THE PAIN DETECTIVE

Recent Titles in
The Praeger Series on Contemporary Health and Living

THE PAIN DETECTIVE
EVERY ACHE TELLS A STORY

Understanding How Stress and Emotional Hurt Become Chronic Physical Pain

HILLEL M. FINESTONE, M.D.

The Praeger Series on Contemporary Health and Living
Julie Silver, M.D., Series Editor

PRAEGER
An Imprint of ABC-CLIO, LLC

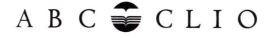

A B C 🌐 C L I O

Santa Barbara, California • Denver, Colorado • Oxford, England

Library of Congress Cataloging-in-Publication Data

Finestone, Hillel M.
    The pain detective : every ache tells a story : understanding how
stress and emotional hurt become chronic physical pain / Hillel M. Finestone.
        p. cm. — (Praeger series on contemporary health and living)
    Includes bibliographical references and index.
    ISBN 978-0-313-35993-4 (hard copy : alk. paper) — ISBN 978-0-313-35994-1 (e-book)
1. Pain—Diagnosis. 2. Chronic diseases. 3. Pain—Psychological aspects. I. Title. II. Series:
Praeger series on contemporary health and living.
    [DNLM: 1. Pain—diagnosis. 2. Chronic Disease. 3. Pain—psychology.
4. Pain—therapy. 5. Stress, Psychological—complications. WL 704 F4955p 2009]
RB127.F565   2009
616'.0472—dc22   2009016488

13   12   11   10   09   1   2   3   4   5

This book is also available on the World Wide Web as an eBook.
Visit www.abc-clio.com for details.

ABC-CLIO, LLC
130 Cremona Drive, P.O. Box 1911
Santa Barbara, California 93116-1911

This book is printed on acid-free paper ∞

Manufactured in the United States of America

This book is dedicated to the memory of my late father David Finestone. His life was guided by his conscience.

CONTENTS

SERIES FOREWORD

Over the past 100 years, there have been incredible medical breakthroughs that have prevented or cured illness in billions of people and helped many more improve their health while living with chronic conditions. A few of the most important 20th-century discoveries include antibiotics, organ transplants and vaccines. The twenty-first century has already heralded important new treatments including such things as a vaccine to prevent human papillomavirus from infecting and potentially leading to cervical cancer in women. Polio is on the verge of being eradicated worldwide, making it only the second infectious disease behind smallpox to ever be erased as a human health threat.

In this series, experts from many disciplines share with readers important and updated medical knowledge. All aspects of health are considered including subjects that are disease specific and preventive medical care. This information will help individuals to improve their health as well as researchers to determine where there are gaps in our current knowledge and policy makers to assess the most pressing needs in healthcare. Dr. Finestone has authored a very personal yet informative book on pain. You will enjoy his insights and practical approach to a complex problem.

Series Editor Julie K. Silver, M.D.
Assistant Professor
Harvard Medical School
Department of Physical Medicine and Rehabilitation

ACKNOWLEDGMENTS

I would like to thank my wife, Linda, and my children, Elana, Benji, and Danielle, for always supporting my writing endeavors. Domenica Ricottilli typed the first drafts and provided the proof that this book could really happen. Huguette Houle converted my scrawl into real text. Gloria Baker was my research associate and in-hospital editor. Linda Greene-Finestone and Dvorah Finestone polished up the manuscript. Shya Finestone provided trivia facts. Many thanks to my mother; Ma—you are in the book.

I'm eternally grateful to Dr. Julie Silver, who first recognized this book's possibilities. Deborah Carvalko was an able editor. Michael Levine, an entertainment lawyer, has encouraged my writing initiatives over the years.

Most of all, I thank my patients, who have inspired me and shown me how healing is a complex yet rewarding process.

INTRODUCTION

As a physiatrist or a specialist in physical medicine and rehabilitation (these terms are synonyms), I have the unique privilege to see people who are experiencing painful conditions. Patients arrive in my office experiencing pain in their neck, back, arms, legs, or knees, and sometimes the pain is from "my head to my toes." They walk, limp, ride buses, cars, and wheelchairs. They have difficulty finding a parking spot on the crowded streets or hospital lot and may get lost in the health center corridors because of the difficult-to-read signs and arrows. Eventually they do make it to my office. They worry about what is going to happen within my four walls, about whether I'll be helpful or whether their street-parked vehicle will have a parking ticket affixed to it when their appointment is over. They are often tired, as their previous night's sleep, and their sleep the night before that, was poor. They wonder whether I'll be kind or tough or judgmental. But one point is clear: they seek relief from their suffering.

My patients are referred by their family doctors or other medical specialists such as neurologists, orthopedic surgeons, anesthetists, rheumatologists, neurosurgeons, or internists. Sometimes the referral note is detailed, and on other occasions it says "chronic low back pain, please see." I would like more information, but it doesn't always arrive with the patient.

Most patients want to get better, some want validation of their pain, and others feel they can't be helped but feel obligated to show up. They usually know they are coming to see a "specialist," but they often have never heard of a *physiatrist,* and they couldn't care less. They want relief, be it in the form of a pill, a salve, a solution, or an electrical device. Some are desperate, and some are calm. Some clutch papers provided to them by government agencies, insurance companies, workers' compensation boards or their own notes (up to 100 pages long). Some have binders of information, and others have consulted multiple Web sites. Most try to remember their stories without any papers at all.

They come with members of their family, former spouses, lovers, union representatives, translators, or friends, "so I won't forget what you said,

Dr. Finestone. She always says I never tell her anything about what the doctor told me." They slowly or briskly walk down the hall. They rub their necks and backs or remain perfectly still. Some are wearing long leg braces, remnants of a distant polio outbreak in the Philippines or Russia. Some limp in because one side of their body is partially paralyzed by the effects of a stroke. A cane or walker may be by their side or in front of them. There is no specific body build or feature that describes the person who is experiencing pain. My patients are all unique in their own physical, psychological, spiritual, and social ways. They are like snowflakes; no two are the same. That is what makes each day so interesting and sometimes so tough.

My patients usually arrive with hope, but sometimes they feel hopeless. Closer or farther away from their skin's surface, an ache is waiting to be soothed, massaged, or expunged. They seek a solution, a plan of attack. They seek relief from episodic or unending pain. They may want to discuss a worn clipping from their hometown newspaper that details some new or old treatment. Ultimately, however, the person in pain suffers and wants to be heard.

The person in pain clutches his back and moans when sitting down or silently walks toward the examining table. Each person in pain tells a different story. He was fine until one day a chair broke or cabinets toppled onto his head. Or, she suffered for years, slowly noticing increasing low back pain, which changed from light fists tapping to daggers thrusting in and out of her flesh.

I listen to their stories. I probe. I ask questions that sometimes wander away from the description of the pain or how it happened. "Why do you need to know about my divorce?" they ask. "I'm here for my pain." Sometimes I'm not exactly sure why I ask a particular question, but most of the time I'm trying to peer, bit by bit, into the soul of the problem. I'm trying the expose the festering wound of emotional and physical hurt. Pain doesn't kill; it maims. Feelings seem to ignite it, and it seems to ignite feelings.

Sometimes it's as easy as "move the mouse from your right hand to your left, slow down on the computer work, and your arm will get better." Dr. Finestone has figured out the problem. But, most of the time, it just doesn't work like that. There is no neat beginning, middle, or end. Many times, I see people after a crisis. Their car was hit from behind while they were driving to work. Their neck pain then escalated to a point where it became difficult to bear. They seek medical attention and somehow get to my office, frequently after a broken bone, torn nerve or ripped rotator cuff muscle has been "ruled out." The terrain starts shifting. The family doctor is wondering, "is this real or . . . what? What is going on? If the problem remains or worsens, he or she will then contact me, asking for advice on how to manage the particular pain problem.

Psychology and sociology are always important in medicine, but retrieving or revealing their key components—those that are important to "figuring out" the person's pain—is my holy grail. This is the "mind-body connection," which must be discovered, mined, and nurtured. Under the right circumstances, much success can be achieved when the mind and body are treated simultaneously, parts of a larger whole. This book tries to explain the complex relationships among mind, body, and pain, via the exploration of clinical journeys my patients and I have taken together.

I knew I had chosen the right title for this book when after about 20 minutes of struggling through a patient's set of painful circumstances—the hows, the whens, the timing, the severity, the burning, the job descriptions, and the mental states—my patient paused. "As a doctor, I guess you're like a detective, Dr. Finestone." I believe she was beginning to understand that many clinical conditions are complicated and involved; the patient and doctor may have to retrieve clues and key bits of information to create a whole diagnostic picture. It's like a detective trying to crack a murder or arson case. It may require sifting through the dust, ashes, and remains of the physical body and the social and psychological mind; uncovering clues that can lead to a life of less pain, of greater fulfillment. Detectives don't solve every case they take on, and I certainly can't help every person who consults me. But I sure as hell try to.

The Pain Detective. As the title suggests, every ache and every person in pain does tell a story. These are the stories of the heroes, the heroines, the tragicomics, the wanderers, the confused, the person on the street and those crying into their beer, scotch, or wine. My patients and I stumble to find the meaning of their pain and what's behind their pain. I will tell you, the reader, what is going on in my head while many diagnoses are being considered and what medical science can offer. When my patients and I find medical clues, key pain-related factors or some small point initially thought to be mundane that helps propel us forward, we have a much better shot at solving the pain problem. It's tough, sometimes fatiguing work. My patients and I may end up in blind alleys, at forks in the road and situations where we both have to take that therapeutic leap into a place that may be initially uncomfortable. But the rewards are great, and the journeys are always worth taking.

The stories in this book are true, but they have been changed and modified so that my patients cannot be identified. Sometimes I have grouped various characteristics, behaviors, and outcomes of a number of patients in order to make a specific point. A few cases have also been melded into one to better illustrate a particular treatment or diagnostic principle.

This book is written for people who are currently experiencing some type of pain, those who have been in pain in the past, and all those who are curious about mind-body interactions and their roles in the experience of pain. The chapters also provide insight into the doctor-patient relationship, sometimes with an element of humor as usually, I'd rather laugh than cry. I want you to know how some doctors reason out a problem and what tools are often at their disposal. There are many ways to handle a particular medical problem, and, as I point out, it is often not easy being a patient. There are often so many opinions and so little time—four therapists, five treatment plans. That's just the way it is.

I believe that medical students and doctors, as well as my so important colleagues in physical therapy, occupational therapy, kinesiology, massage therapy, chiropractic, orthotics and prosthetics, osteopathy, social work, and psychology will also benefit from the approaches my patients and I have taken together. Lawyers who deal in personal injury, vocational counselors, social security personnel, insurance adjustors, and those who work with people with disabilities will also likely enjoy the real interactions discussed. Security, police, and army-affiliated individuals will recognize relevant issues, as well. Pain crosses so many borders and boundaries. No one is immune from its reaches. Understanding it better can help us understand ourselves, or maybe it's the other way around.

These "pain stories" are sometimes disturbing, frequently exciting, and often uplifting. They will not lead the reader to the only true path to pain relief, because there never is one exclusive way. These chapters and the stories within them will, however, provide the reader with new ideas and connections. Readers may see pieces of themselves or others somewhere within a particular story and thus be able to help devise recovery plans for themselves, patients, friends, or clients. That is my goal. I hope that these stories will inspire some to take charge of their health and pain issues. Everyone knows that is not easy to do. But it is worth it and it can be done.

The next chapter describes some basic principles of pain, acute and chronic. Subsequently, I move on to chapters that focus on particular themes. Pain related to work, pain and abuse, pain and fatigue, pain and exercise, the risk factors for pain, pain and alcohol, pain and relationships, stress/anxiety and pain, pain and the active person, and pain and fibromyalgia syndrome are some of the subjects covered. Throughout I offer my sometimes tangential thoughts concerning clinical pet peeves, preferred treatments and medications, and the disappointing realities of the "pain industry." I often refer to an appended one-page sheet called the "pain explanation and treatment diagram." I use this tool in my medical practice, and my patients and I fill it out together. My hope is that, after reading this book, the person in pain will be able to complete the sheet with his or her doctor, thus gaining better insight and understanding into his or her own particular pain issues.

Let the stories begin.

1

MUSCULOSKELETAL PAIN, STRESS, WOUND HEALING, AND MIND–BODY RELATIONSHIPS: A NEW PERSPECTIVE

Few people in this world have not experienced pain in one form or another. An ankle sprain after a fall, with swelling and pain that last two minutes, two hours, two months, or even two years; the slow steady development of extreme visual sensitivity when looking at bright lights, nausea, vomiting, and an intolerable, mind-numbing migraine headache; low back pain that grumbles on day after day, worsening after a three-hour car ride, a prolonged computer keyboard session, or too much Sunday afternoon gardening. These are common human events that can lead to suffering and despondency.

Pain deprives people of establishing relationships and keeps them from enjoying family or work-related events. It can socially isolate both those experiencing pain and their loved ones or caregivers.

Too many people suffer pain in silence. Chronic pain, often defined as pain experienced on a frequent to continuous basis for longer than three months, is too common. Chronic low back pain and chronic neck pain are major sources of hardship and disability in society.

Billions of dollars per year are expended on pain treatments, primarily physical and pharmaceutical related. Not enough is spent on understanding those who are experiencing the pain, the circumstances under which they live, their backgrounds, their stresses and their actual lives. Certainly, many psychologists and sociologists study pain, and many excellent research projects have resulted from their work. However, integration of their findings into mainstream medicine is lacking. When you take into account disability and unemployment insurance, social security benefits, government welfare payments required for painful conditions, legal fees, costs associated with car accidents and workers' compensation benefits, the price paid out in the name of pain climbs to a high peak. Hundreds of millions of dollars are dispensed yearly in Canada, the United States, Europe, Australia, Asia, South America and other jurisdictions where financial benefits for disability are available. We need to better understand the multitude of factors that contribute to these major costs. This, in turn, will contribute to the alleviation of people's painful conditions.

Musculoskeletal pain (pain related to or emanating from muscles, ligaments, and joints, like low back or neck pain) is a huge cause of suffering, sadness, and inactivity. It is a major focus of this book as I explain the injuries and conditions that can involve and affect these parts of the body's anatomy. Real stories about medical cases that I have had the honor to assess over the years are recounted. Musculoskeletal pain occurs after an injury such as a fall, after a long run, after a long bout at the computer and sometimes it is so hard to ascertain how it began. This book tries to help the reader "figure it out," as the patient in the first story (Chapter 2) does.

In the next sections I discuss how pain is experienced, where pain's body pathways are located, and how the mind and body interact in the experience of pain. I cite relevant scientific articles about these subjects, particularly articles on stress and wound healing.

How Does One Feel Pain?

"Pain is all in the mind, Dr. Finestone" were the words once uttered to me by a chairman of a university department of physical medicine and rehabilitation. True, without a brain we probably would not feel any pain. The good doctor was trying, I suppose, to impress upon me that all of the focus on treatment to cure or heal the pain in the arm, leg, neck, or whatever body part was somewhat futile, especially if the pain was longstanding.

My colleague is right, and he is very wrong. Treatment of pain must indeed focus on the mind, as so many of the stories and cases in this book attest. However, the injured part(s) needs to be attended to as well. Sometimes a "chronic" pain is that way only because a particular physical issue, such as poor blood glucose control in a diabetic patient or the need for a rigorous strengthening program, has not been addressed. A proper diagnosis that at least explains which body tissues are involved, not just the diagnosis of "chronic pain," is always needed. An accurate concurrent assessment of the psychological and sociological events surrounding the case may be equally important in solving the pain puzzle.

Pain seems to serve a number of purposes. One appreciates how a sudden injury to the tips of one's fingers from touching the electrical or gas burner causes sudden sharp pain. The pain is a clear warning that localized damage is occurring, and the response is to pull the hand away, as quickly as possible. Some call this fast pain. Slow pain, the burning ache surrounding the general injury, may induce muscles to become firm or contract, encouraging immobilization and allowing time for the injury to heal. As the pain message leaves pain receptors in our skin, it follows a complex pathway along a sensory nerve (akin to an electrical wire) to the spinal cord (a neurological way station housed in the bony vertebrae or "backbones" where messages are hurled up and down in milliseconds) and finally to many locations of the brain. The relay stations in the spinal cord and brain are described as pain gates. Ultimately, the conscious mind interprets the incoming signal and bam! the finger is boomeranging away from the heat source, the sharp knife blade, or any other painful stimulus.

Referred pain can be understood as pain experienced as if it derived from a particular body part, such as the big toe, when the problem is actually somewhere along the pain's pathway. Examples include compression of the sciatic nerve, buried deep in one's buttock, by a fat wallet in one's back pocket or the pinching of a nerve root in the back by a disc herniation. Examination of the painful big toe will not provide the nurse or doctor with any useful information at all because the problem is actually a number of feet away.

If a pain pathway is open too long, circuits can become hypersensitive, and the person continues to experience pain after the stimulus is long gone. Endorphins (substances produced by the body) may block the receptors of slow chronic pain just as morphine, a narcotic drug sometimes prescribed for pain relief, does. Other drugs are designed to work at different levels, such as on neurotransmitters, the chemicals that pass nerve messages throughout the brain and spinal cord. Drugs like ASA work on inflammation in the body, and acetaminophen acts in the brain to decrease the febrile response as well as the sensation of pain. Aspirin and other nonsteroidal anti-inflammatory drugs, such as ibuprofen or naproxen, may lead to stomach bleeding, whereas acetaminophen does not have this side effect. Obviously, you must consult your doctor and/or pharmacist about your pain medications and learn about the pros, cons, side effects, and possible interactions with other drugs you may be taking.

That was a very short primer on some aspects of pain. Major books and monographs have been written describing the intricacies and the mechanisms of pain. Diagnostic and rating scales have been constructed, such as the rating of one's pain as a scale from 1 to 10. I will never forget one particular patient to whom I explained that a rating of 10 essentially meant that one was being burned alive, with sharp knives probing every skin crease at the same time. Although she was well groomed, was sitting quietly, and had told me that she was still working in a management position, she still rated her pain as 10. I learned that the meaning and interpretation of any pain can be very different according to the individual, his or her circumstances, and many other factors. This observation was actually one of the reasons why I sought to find out what those other factors could be. This quest never really ends. The fact that my patient rated her pain as 10 was likely a reflection of the tremendous physical and emotional distress she was experiencing. To her, the pain was unbearable, and she was the only person who was experiencing her suffering. Having a better understanding of why one's pain seems to be insurmountable and then receiving appropriate help is the only way for recovery and pain relief to occur. The stories to come detail the factors required to achieve positive pain and life outcomes. More scientific thought is required now before we get to those stories.

MUSCULOSKELETAL PAIN: SOME NEW THOUGHTS

There are many models to describe how fast pain becomes slow pain and how there may not be any pain coming from the originally involved part, such as the back or neck. The injured musculoskeletal tissue is thereafter bypassed, and the pain is deemed to be a product of disordered, irrational pain fibers, spinal cord highways, and brain stations. There are a number of painful conditions of the back, neck, and limbs that do represent some type of poor function of the central nervous system (brain and spinal cord). Reflex sympathetic dystrophy and neuropathic pain due to head or nerve trauma are fairly common examples of "pain gone amok" where doctors have trouble pinpointing one organ or body part as the primary focus of the painful condition. Pain, swelling, redness, dryness, contracture, and hypersensitivity to touch may be signs and symptoms of these problems.

However, there are many other painful and longstanding chronic conditions that don't necessarily emanate from an injured or aberrantly firing nerve, spinal cord, or brain. Over the years, I have evaluated thousands of patients, and I have come to appreciate that there are other ideas about musculoskeletal pain. Injured muscles and ligaments can cause prolonged pain, as well. Myofascial pain, musculoligamentous pain, strain pain, and the "tension myositis" pain described by Dr. John Sarno are all worthwhile terms that reflect what may be going on at the level of the muscles and ligaments when they are a source of ongoing pain.

Scientific literature has focused on pain gates, pain transmission pathways, and other central nervous system ways of thinking about pain; however, there are also many very interesting articles on peripheral wound healing and recovery from injury, in both animals and humans. This literature is extremely intriguing, and has enabled me to better appreciate the particular effects that mood and emotions may have on injured tissues, skeletal muscle, and even recovery from surgery.

The mind and the body have been studied in many unique ways, linking the experience of stress or anxiety with:

1. a delayed ability to recover from a skin or leg wound and;
2. a deleterious effect on skeletal muscle.

Skeletal muscle is the sometimes thin, occasionally bulky material that gives you, me, and the musclebound woman on the beach much of our shape. Skeletal muscle is also what we eat when we're munching on a tasty charbroiled steak. This may sound disgusting, but it's the truth. It is skeletal muscle that often gets injured, either in the substance of the muscle or farther downstream where the muscle becomes a tendon and then attaches into the bone. Injuries occur while running, walking, sitting at our desks, lifting boxes, cleaning out the garage, or just closing a low filing cabinet drawer.

I talk a lot about musculoskeletal injury and related pain via my patients' experiences in this book. In a scientific article published by the *Clinical Journal of Pain,* I wrote about how stress induces physiological changes and how these changes may relate to the experience of chronic musculoskeletal pain.[1] In one experiment, a bunch of stressed mice were compared to a nonstressed group. How do you stress a mouse? The investigators say you "restrain" them, that is, you put them in a tube so they can't move. That's stressful. The other group of mice was allowed to roam about and eat whenever they wanted to. The experimenters then created a small wound on the back of both groups of animals and observed how long it took the wound to heal over. What was the result? As you may have suspected, it took longer for the wounds to heal in the stressed mice than in the nonstressed mice.

The investigators also wanted to try to determine what factor(s) led to this difference in healing. They thought it might be a result of the fact that during a stressful reaction of any type, the chemical cortisol is secreted by our adrenal glands, the same glands that pump out adrenaline when we're excited, frightened, or responding to some form of danger. Cortisol is needed by our bodies to mount an effective stress response. It also has anti-inflammatory properties that decreases the body's inflammation reaction to a small degree. Inflammatory responses are needed to fight infection and to control and repair wounds. Having too much cortisol due to excessive stress could, however, induce a situation in which not enough inflammation is occurring and, therefore, wounds are not being healed.

The investigators then gave the stressed mice a drug that blocked the mice's ability to "pick up" the cortisol. The thought was that this would, in effect, block the effect of excessive cortisol produced in the stressed mice. What happened? The wound healing in the stressed mice reverted to a normal healing time. The message is that stress affects wound healing by impairing the immune system. Stress "revs up" the cortisol response and decreases the inflammatory response, and the wound takes longer to heal.

Thus, the case to be made with us humans is that if we're very stressed, because of work, home, love life, or childhood factors, there is an increased chance at the time of our injury that we will have a harder time healing and therefore recovering. This makes a lot of sense to me and to my patients, as well. It nicely connects the mind and the body and allows us to think about musculoskeletal treatment in a nonthreatening, holistic manner. It helps my patients and me to stop blaming stress as the sole cause of the problem and to focus on a combined mind-body recovery approach.

There are a number of other studies that look at this stress/wound healing model. In one study, by the brilliant Dr. Janice Kiecolt-Glaser of Ohio State University and her colleagues, stressed caregivers taking care of their cognitively impaired loved ones were studied. Their stress and anxiety were scored, and they then received a small skin wound, which the investigators followed through its stages of healing. What happened? Basically the same events as in the mice: the stressed caregivers could not heal their skin wounds as fast as lesser-stressed or nonstressed subjects. Dr. Kiecolt-Glaser's group's research on marital stress and wound healing showed that healing took two days longer in couples with high levels of hostility than in couples whose hostility levels appeared low. In addition, wounds took a day longer to heal after marital arguments than after initial supportive positive discussion. Of course, the correlations were not perfect. Any theory in science or medicine rarely is perfect, but the research provides us with much food for thought and practice. Other findings include delayed healing of wounds created in the hard palate of dental students stressed by school examinations and delayed healing of wounds created on the nondominant arm of people with relatively low levels of anger control. Still another study indicated that writing about a personal, upsetting experience resulted in smaller wounds that healed quicker than did writing about trivial matters. One interpretation of these findings was that expressing emotions in writing leads to lower stress levels. These lower stress levels are, in turn, reflected in the biochemical environment of a subject's body, and they therefore facilitate wound healing. The overall message: psychological stress—often defined as the threat of damage, either real or imagined, frequently related to conflict and frustration—affects our ability to heal from an injury such as a wound.

For years scientists have written about other body responses to threats, including increases in heart rate, blood pressure, blood sugar, muscle tension, and respiration rate. Wound-related impairments can now be added to the overall musculoskeletal pain picture. Let's now look at how muscle may react to stress.

In a study in a laboratory setting, the back muscles of stressed subjects were shown to be more contracted than those of unstressed subjects while doing lifting tasks. Women were more affected than men. The message here is that if you're feeling tense (i.e., worried, fretting, or afraid), your body's skeletal muscle is also tense. The muscle and ligament chemistry is affected. Muscles contract more, and the thought is that tight, contracted muscles also increase spine compression and you then hurt more. As I explain in Chapter 11, most of our muscles are not designed to be held in a constant state of contraction for prolonged periods. Rather, they should be contracting and relaxing intermittently. As other stories demonstrate, our recognizing obvious or hidden thoughts, stresses, secrets, and lies may allow our chronically contracted muscles to relax, open up, and welcome the beneficial effects of exercise. Ultimately, the hurt is lessened, and pain is reduced or eliminated.

Mood affects so many medical outcomes. Surgeons have written that a depressed person may have a poorer and longer recovery after any type of surgery than a nondepressed person. Many theories can be put forth to indicate why this may be so. A few demeaning and usually, in my experience, untrue reasons include these: (1) depressed people are less motivated to recover, and (2) depressed people complain more for any given pain experience, and that is a major part of the delayed recovery. These are unfounded, generally boorish comments. Obviously, there are other ways to look at the issues of surgery and mood.

The findings regarding the immune system, wound healing, and excessive muscle contraction shine new light on the depression-delayed recovery data.

Depressed people may have impaired wound healing or impaired skeletal muscle function, or both. These factors, and multiple others, may explain some aspects of their delayed recovery. In fact, the authors of a study about hernia repair noted that psychological stress slows wound healing by impairing the inflammatory response and the matrix degradation process in the wound immediately following surgery. In another study, patients undergoing gallbladder surgery were provided with relaxation techniques; lower cortisol levels and less surgical wound redness (erythema) were noted postoperatively. It is always convenient to implicate purely psychological factors such as stress, anxiety, and depression as the sole reasons for someone's chronic pain or delayed recovery. They rarely are the sole cause. However, the mind and the body do work pretty closely together, and they form fairly powerful connections that can ultimately be quite harmful. The trials and judgments of "regular people" with regard to their pain issues are detailed in subsequent chapters.

Studies about slaughtered animals popped up in my colleague's Google search when we were investigating stress, wound healing, and recovery from injury topics. The results were fascinating. Veterinarians suspected that something about how animals were handled before being slaughtered was affecting the quality of the meat, which, as mentioned previously, is skeletal muscle. Meat could be affected negatively by being either pale and soft or dark and firm. Scientists deduced that longer and rougher transportation, that is, stressful handling, produced these negative qualities of meat after slaughter. This information was intriguing to my colleagues and me because it seemed to indicate, once again, that stress, anxiety, and worry directly affect not only the brain and the spinal cord but also the musculoskeletal system. In the slaughtered animals' case, the skeletal muscles were negatively affected. Too high lactic acid concentrations or changes in electrical conductivity were noted, but it was not possible to pinpoint exactly which stress factor led to the production of poor meat quality. Australian beef producers noted similar findings in their meat. They decided that herding cattle using cowboys and horses produced a higher-quality product than did herding accomplished with noisy, stress-inducing helicopters.

Although the animal studies may seem to be coming out of left field, I think they have relevance to those of us who belong to the human species. After all, we are not that different from our fellow creatures in the animal kingdom. And the message for us humans? Something in the way we behave and react affects the biochemistry and the physiology of our muscles and ligaments. We can further imagine, therefore, that changes in our muscles and ligaments may be happening not only after a frank injury such as a fall or fracture but also throughout the day when we're thinking, stressing, bemoaning, disappointing, overachieving, mourning, dreaming, arguing, talking on the phone. . . . The list is endless.

This information on wound healing and skeletal muscle physiology is really no surprise to cardiologists and people with cardiovascular disease. Research has particularly focused on mind-body issues and the health of the heart.

Proper diet and stress reduction, achieved via various techniques including exercise and meditation, has been shown to, for instance, transform narrowed coronary arteries (the tubes that feed blood into the actual heart muscle) into wider ones; people then experience less chest pain and greater exercise tolerance. Musculoskeletal medicine seems to be a little farther behind cardiovascular medicine, probably because there are fewer tests available to show musculoskeletal injury or abnormal function. It is therefore harder to show how muscle and ligament tissues recover after stress is reduced, changes are made to the work site, and healthier lifestyles are adopted. I describe, however, what tests doctors order to diagnose muscle and ligament problems throughout the stories contained in this book.

Dr. Hans Selye's pivotal work on "fight-or-flight" reactions pioneered research about the stress response. Dr. Selye determined that the fight-or-flight response (whereby one flees or mounts an aggressive response to a threat) could be triggered by psychological factors as well as by physical threats. He laid the groundwork for researchers to determine that the stress we experience and our reactions to it play an integral role in health and disease. The autonomic nervous system—the particular system that works behind the scenes, keeping our hearts beating and maintaining blood vessel tone, even when we are not aware of these functions—jumps to the front of the line in moments of crisis, such as when we need to run away from a bear that we meet suddenly on a stroll in the forest or in times of war or trauma. So the autonomic nervous system is a very important one, but if it is triggered too often, excessive muscle contraction, blood flow changes, anxiety, exhaustion, and pain may result. More food for thought about the roles of mind and body in perpetuating or initiating a painful condition. Accelerating your vehicle in order to pass another vehicle is fine, but keeping the gas pedal slammed to the floor will undoubtedly lead to dysfunction. Mick Jagger describes this relationship in the song "Driving Too Fast" on the Rolling Stones' album *A Bigger Bang*. Stress, excessive tension, life events involving families, money, jobs—all can lead to a chronic painful condition or a situation whereby you may need to "hang on to the wheel, I think you're going to crash."

In the upcoming chapters, I recount and discuss various clinical cases. I provide an accurate description of how a particular case evolved and how the diagnosis was made. In my practice, I often ask about psychological and social issues, ergonomic factors, the role of sleep and exercise, and habits such as smoking and drinking alcohol. I use the responses to weave my patient and me through a treatment model that incorporates some of the described scientific principles on wound and musculoskeletal recovery.

A diagnostic and treatment model that illustrates the multitude of factors that can affect the health of musculoskeletal tissues, particularly muscles and ligaments, is provided in the Appendix at the back of this volume. This "Pain Explanation and Treatment" diagram, which is often talked about in the course of the stories and cases discussed, nicely summarizes just how complex the science of treatment of and recovery from a painful condition is. I often use and refer to the concepts talked about in this chapter to help my patients through their difficult painful times. The diagram helps me to initiate a treatment plan. Of course, there are other models out there, and one should never use a "cookie-cutter" approach with the patient in pain. But the diagram is useful, and the reader can use it, too. The roles of habits, sleep, exercise, ergonomics, and psychological and social factors in hampering, delaying, and perpetuating recovery are the key features of the diagram. By the end of this book, you will be quite familiar with it.

Other models of pain include a psychodynamic model. A colleague of mine relates all of my patients' complaints of pain and stiffness to their childhood miseries. He may indicate that the current pain disability is merely an excuse for the person to avoid work and family responsibilities. Maybe that does happen sometimes, but I don't think that this model is diverse or broad enough to account for all of my patient's pains and difficulties.

There are models that consider the person's propensity to "catastrophize" in the face of a painful experience. Such a person may react very strongly to a particular painful condition, thinking that there is no chance of recovery, that return to work will be impossible, or that disability is inevitable. Those who catastrophize to a strong degree (a rating scale can indicate the degree) are noted to recover more poorly from work-related injuries and arthritic conditions. This is a good model, if somewhat limited, but it fits with many other concepts about pain. Catastrophizing may induce many of the same effects as severe stress and lead to impaired recovery from injury or disease.

Cognitive behavioral models consider treatment in terms of the here and now, that is, they deal with new stresses, anxiety, posttraumatic stress, fears about driving a vehicle, and the fear patients may have of resuming their previous lives. This is a successful model of treatment that works well if relevant past life issues are also discussed, in my opinion. Sometimes the model does not deal with past issues such as abuse (Chapter 9), and then it can become problematic.

Other treatment models focus on coping and accepting the chronic painful condition that the patient may be experiencing. Rehabilitation-oriented multi-disciplinary pain centers have shown excellent success in enabling their clients to increase their physical activity, lighten their moods, and generally engage in activities they may have abandoned years earlier. When this is combined with a personal psychotherapeutic focus, much success can occur.

But let's get back to my—and now our—model. We'll acknowledge but leave the central aspects of pain for others to further dissect and discuss. I have reviewed an incredibly powerful new set of research ideas that relate to the roles that sociology and psychology play in the body's immunology, wound healing and skeletal muscle function. Figure 1.1 is a schematic diagram that summarizes much of the ideas. It demonstrates how circular the problem of chronic pain can become in the form of a feedback loop. Focusing in on the physical and emotional elements of my patients' cases has allowed

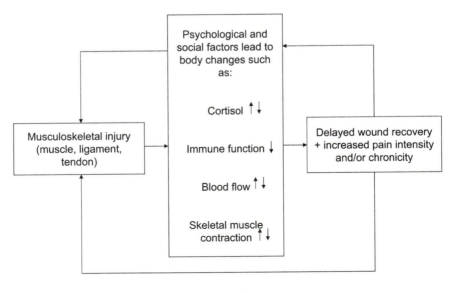

Feedback loop

Figure 1.1. Model of Musculoskeletal Injury and Pain: Mind-Body Interactions.

me to better understand and treat their painful conditions. If you have pain, you may try to assess where it fits into the diagram.

We will learn about the mind-body connection through the true case stories that I will tell. We will discover how powerful the mind can be in determining how we feel and behave and how it can actually affect disease. I now challenge you to read about my patients' journeys and see how a combination of art and science helped improve their musculoskeletal injuries and pain syndromes in a caring and cohesive manner, a manner that incorporated the mind and the body to promote healing and recovery.

Sometimes a shard of glass enters the deep belly of the leg's calf muscle, and the individual feels pain. When the glass is surgically removed the pain dissipates and the muscle heals and returns to normal. In most cases, an episode of back pain resolves without any particular intervention except "I slowed down." Sometimes psychological and social factors from the past, present, or future can affect, influence, or possibly even cause a particular painful condition. We are heading into the real world of science, mind, body, and, occasionally, a bit of faith—faith in ourselves, in the world as it is, and in the ability of doctors and therapists to help with particularly difficult pain conditions.

One thing I know for sure is this: if someone says he or she possesses all the answers, it is clear that that person doesn't possess much. Knowing about some of the science that ticks away within us can be very important in understanding ourselves and some, but not all, of our pains. This chapter has not explained everything about musculoskeletal injury and pain, but some unique perspectives have been revealed, and I use most of them in the stories that follow. The science is woven into the art of medicine. It is the combination of the science and the art, the mind and the body, the cold hard data and the abstract concepts, that makes a case, and therefore a human being, come alive. I will be your guide, your pain detective, as we look at the mysterious world of musculoskeletal pain.

NOTE

1. H. M. Finestone, A. Alfeeli, and W. A. Fisher, "Stress-Induced Physiologic Changes as a Basis for the Biopsychosocial Model of Chronic Musculoskeletal Pain: A New Theory?," *Clinical Journal of Pain* 24, no. 9 (2008): 767–775.

2

She Figured It Out: A Case of Back Pain

Back pain is ubiquitous in today's society. Who hasn't experienced some kind of back pain at one time or another? Statistics say that sometime during our lives an episode of back pain will occur and more than 90 percent of the time, it will resolve. But that's a group statistic, part of the "epidemiology" or "health care science" of back pain. That's for a "simple" case of back pain, one without complications, without serious side effects and without major problems. The statistics certainly change according to the type of back diagnosis and whether surgery is required. Age also may make a difference in recovery. Older people find it harder to bounce back from any medical issue. Back pain in the presence of other diseases, such as diabetes, which can sicken nerves and blood vessels, may take longer to heal. Smokers seem to experience more back pain than nonsmokers. Smokers' injured tissues may not recover as well because smoking plugs up blood vessels. Blood, which carries healing materials such as red and white blood cells and oxygen, is less able to reach the damaged muscles and ligaments. Other toxic effects of cigarette smoke could be involved as well.

Issues such as feelings, emotions, and life events, may bridge the mind and the body and play a role in the diagnosis and treatment of back pain. That is actually a large part of my practice—finding out information, hunting for clues that may reveal the real source of my patients' suffering. Let's explore Ann's case and find out what some of those issues may be.

Ann was referred by her family doctor because of "persisting pain, thoracolumbar [chest and low back area], x-rays show some degenerative changes, active female, please assess." As I walked into the examination room, I saw that Ann was thin, muscular, and fit-looking. The date of birth at the top of the chart told me that she was 28 years old.

I try to capture a quick overview of the person I'm seeing: age, right- or left-handed, single or married (first time, second time, third time). Ann was divorced. Number of children? Two, ages three and six. Are they healthy? Yes. I'm still not wholly comfortable asking about sexual orientation up front, although I do think about the issue. If I think it's relevant, then I'll ask about it later. Is the person working? Not working? On disability benefits?

Ann's eyebrows arched a bit with this line of questioning. "Anything the matter?" I asked. "Well, to tell you the truth, I'm not really sure why I need to talk about my kids or my marriage—after all, I'm here for my back pain." I explained that I wanted to know a bit about her and her life. I reasoned that if someone had, for instance, a child with Down syndrome (a genetic problem that can affect growth, intellect, and personal independence, among other issues) and was required to regularly bathe the child, even when the child was older, back pain could ensue or just not heal well once it had begun. The forces on the back exerted by carrying the child would be potentially hard on the muscles, ligaments, joints, discs, and even nerves of the back. Similarly, marital status can explain some of life's tensions. For example, going through a divorce is potentially quite stressful, and stress can have a negative impact on the healing and recovery of injured back structures as well (as mentioned in Chapter 1). I indicated to Ann that if I have some idea about these issues, I feel better able to understand the pain story that follows. Ann seemed to accept my remarks, which were uttered in complete sincerity.

Ann lived in an apartment and worked as a retail store manager. Her life was busy. Her two kids lived with her most of the time. They moved to Dad's apartment every second weekend. Her problem was back pain.

In the field of medicine and probably the rest of life, history is key. History is the patient's story, the sequence of life events associated with or causing a particular set of symptoms, signs, or behaviors. Sometimes I joke that for a female I should change the term history to "herstory." Her story was what I really did need to know. Patients often think that medical tests are what make the diagnosis. However, we still teach in medical school that patients' histories will yield the most diagnostic fruit, rather than the physical examination and any x-rays or blood tests that may be ordered. Yes, sometimes we doctors may be too quick to go straight to those fancy tests like the MRI (magnetic resonance imaging, a test that uses magnetic forces to provide very clear body images). We know we shouldn't, but we feel compelled to use technology.

Ann's low back pain had started about three years earlier. There was no known fall, twist, or car accident that she could recall. The pain was local but involved a fairly broad area about one foot long in the middle of her low back. It was often worse in the morning, when she would particularly feel "stiffness" in the area. If she moved or flexed in a certain way, she could feel a kind of "unlocking" or "unzipping" of her back, and the pain would become dramatically reduced. If she "cracked" her back in this manner one or two times per day, the pain would lessen.

But pain was still present throughout the day. Housecleaning, lifting, bending, and particularly bathing her kids aggravated her back pain. "I don't think a young person like me should be feeling this way. It's annoying." Ann wasn't saying she could not cope. She said that she could get through a retail sales day, "but some days are worse than others." When new shipments came in and she had to remove the clothing from the boxes and hang up or fold them, pain in the back would worsen, particularly that night. Could I help? That is what she wanted to know.

More history was needed.

"Are you experiencing any pain down your leg?" (seen in nerve root problems or disc herniations).

"No."

"Any numbness or tingling in your legs?" (also experienced in cases of nerve injury at the level of the back).

"No."

"Are you having any trouble peeing or pooing ? are you ever unable to hold onto your urine or stool? are you ever incontinent?" (possible signs of nerve or spinal cord or even brain problems).

"No, I'm fine with those."

"Can you exercise?"

"Yes, I go on a treadmill three to four times per week. I have no more time for anything else, Dr. Finestone."

I then went over the PQRSTU system of diagnosing a painful condition (as mentioned in Chapter 4): **p**ain, its **q**uality, **r**adiation, **s**everity, **t**iming, and **u**nder what circumstances. Her aching back pain was fairly focal, did not radiate down her leg, was worse with activity and was not constant. Hmmm. . . .

The detective work began. What was going on? Was this a bone problem, a muscle problem, a nerve problem, a cancer, an arthritic disease, an infection? Each question I asked was aimed at searching out the "answer" to the back pain. And yet, most medical texts tell the doctor not to always be too aggressive in figuring out the source of back pain, as it is so common and usually goes away on its own. This is true, but I was the consultant, and the pain hadn't gone away.

So far, nothing was sticking out as a major diagnosis. If this were cancer, it likely would have reared its ugly head in the form of some kind of weakness, loss of feeling, or increased pain earlier. This pain was three years old. Other types of back pain, such as an arthritic type like ankylosing spondylitis, would have appeared in a different way, such as the patient's experiencing neck and shoulder stiffness. None of the serious "red flags," symptoms or signs that mean something serious is happening (discussed in greater detail in Chapter 9), such as bowel or bladder incontinence, fever, weakness, or history of cancer were present here, thank God, Jesus, Mohammed, and other deities of the world.

Asking about life and social or psychological issues, which I try to casually do, can be tricky. Ann was wondering again why I was not so casually asking about stress, time pressures, work satisfaction. "I'm here for my back," she told me, once again. I explained that all kinds of things, such as stress, unhappiness, and overwork, can affect back muscles and ligaments and that I was just trying to be complete. She grudgingly nodded as if to say, "Okay, let's get on with it."

I was thinking that she was nice, cooperative, and cool, but how would I feel if a stranger were suddenly asking all kinds of personal questions? It takes time to develop a trusting relationship. I wanted to get more information but felt that I had asked enough for now.

Ann was provided with a gown. Occasionally patients are perplexed about the need for one. They inform me that usually they are just asked to "pull up my shirt." To examine the spine properly I need to be able to see its contours, watch how it moves, and perform other maneuvers. A gown that opens at the back is usually the best kind of garment for the purpose because it allows these types of examinations. I left the room, and when I returned, I listened to her heart and chest. When my stethoscope was over her heart, I noted, "It's definitely beating." An ice breaker. She looked puzzled, then nodded, "I get it." I then commenced the musculoskeletal examination, the part that retrieves information from the joints, muscles, and ligaments of the body. I asked her to bend forward and turn. I checked for any tender areas by pressing firmly, with my fingertips, on the muscles lining the spine and over the gluteal (buttock) muscles; not a lot to find, hardly tender. Ann was very flexible, and she could touch the floor with the palms of her hands. She noted, however, some pain referred to that same low back area with most movements.

The neurological exam was comforting. It didn't reveal any weakness. There was no loss of sensation over the spot where I jabbed a disposable, plastic-coated "pin." Reflexes? They were great. Knees and ankles jerked easily with the tap of my hammer just like they're supposed to. Weak or absent reflexes can imply a nerve injury. Bounding, exaggerated reflexes could point to a brain or spinal cord problem.

History, physical examination . . . what's next? The family doctor had faxed me various lab reports and tests. The summary that I wrote on the fax cover sheet was "GMG," my Yiddish slang for "Goornist Mit Goornist," or "nothing with nothing."

However, my review of the radiologist's back x-ray report indicated "something with something." In fact, there was noted to be a bony defect called a "spondylolysis" at the level of the L4, L5 vertebrae, the building blocks of the spine. *Is this x-ray abnormality the source of her pain?* Suddenly my persona converted from a lab-coated doctor into Tevye the milkman in the Broadway play *Fiddler on the Roof.*

On the one hand, as Tevye would say, she had pain for three years, the pain was fairly focal, and certain movements seemed to aggravate it. These signs (information obtained from the physical exam) and symptoms (information provided by the patient) fit with the diagnosis of the spondylolysis.

But, on the other hand, as Tevye would say, the medical textbooks tell us that spondylolysis is a bony defect that develops in a person's teens, often in dancers and gymnasts, and that, therefore, it likely had been present for many years, years during which Ann didn't experience any back pain. Maybe it's just a red herring, a tease, a crack in a wooden beam that's there but will not affect the beam's ability to capably hold up the wall for another hundred years.

Maybe the bony defect is like wrinkles on your face representing some kind of skin breakdown but not causing any kind of problem, pain or otherwise.

On the other, third, alien hand, maybe certain activities or postures "activated" the spondylolytic defect and converted a non-pain-causing, previously "inert" structure into currently a painful condition. "Someone give me guidance," I mumbled to myself. "The medical textbooks rarely cover problems like this."

On the basis of my past clinical experience, however, I knew that Ann's problem was not unique. The general thought process is, "It may not be a painful area, but it could be, and if it is, the person should probably stay away from heavier types of physical activities." Fine advice if you're a lawyer or office worker, but not too helpful if you're a furniture mover, factory worker, or retail store manager who really needs her body to bend and lift and put bread on the table. Like Ann.

I left the room, Ann dressed, and I returned to the examination room to summarize my thoughts and findings. I told Ann about the x-ray findings and their possible explanation of her pain. She had gone for physiotherapy in the past year but felt that it had not helped, and she remained very active. I said that I wanted to order a bone scan, a special type of nuclear medicine bone test. This is what the field of injecting a small amount of radioactive material into the body to detect certain diseases is called. It is sometimes facetiously called "unclear medicine" by those of us in the medical trade because of the rather fuzzy small images that are produced. A bone scan can sometimes show "heat," or increased radioactivity, over the area of a spondylolytic defect, and if it does, it usually means that there may be inflammation due to abnormal movement at the site of the defect. This could give further ammunition to the idea that the spondylolysis was the area of concern.

But I was not convinced. My antennae were up. Ann is tense. Not very introspective, it appeared. Maybe some of the pain was related to this tension.

I recommended that Ann do more flexion-type exercises. Flexion, or bending, is said to aggravate the back to a much lesser extent than extension of the spine, or leaning back. She could do them while on a break, sitting on a chair and leaning forward, trying to bring her head between her knees and touching the backs of her hands on the floor.

Then I talked about ergonomics—the body–machine connection—and the need to place the back in positions that were not painful. Ann agreed to look at how she unpacked boxes, how she stood at the cash. I recommended that she purchase a cushioned mat to stand on as it sometimes helps. I wrote this on a prescription pad so that maybe her employer would pay for it. After all, it was a type of medical device. Ann was a working manager and couldn't delegate much to her fellow employees. Too bad.

We then discussed sleep and how a lack of it can aggravate a painful back. Feeling tired throughout the day doesn't allow one to exercise as one likes, and injuries occur more frequently when one is tired. There is a raft of articles that try to link sleep problems with pain syndromes. I don't always agree with the mechanisms that are discussed, but everyone knows that if you don't sleep well for one to a few nights, you just don't feel "right," and neither do your muscles and bones. We talked about the use of a sleep aid medication, but she wasn't interested. She felt that she slept fairly well. I certainly never try to force a patient to take a sleep medication, but sometimes the issue has to be discussed (discussed more extensively in Chapter 5).

Lastly, I brought up the role of life in general in anyone's back pain. I showed Ann a list of conditions (see Appendix, Pain Explanation and Treatment Diagram) that, in my experience, can aggravate, worsen, or "screw up" anyone's muscle, ligament, neck, back, arm, shoulder, or even toe pain. Adrenaline is squirted into the blood system, leading to excessive sweating, changes in blood flow, and muscle contraction and pain increases. The list expands as grey hairs accumulate on my head: money (not enough of it), problems with kids, marital troubles, a history of physical or sexual abuse, alcoholism (we'll get to these in other stories).

Ann was poker-faced and didn't think any of these were relevant issues, having had a good family life and a fine relationship with her parents and siblings. Yes, there was her failed marriage, but that was in the past.

My role is not to judge. I provide the information. "I'm not saying that your pain is due to some kind of stress or whatever, but as an expert in this area, I'm trying to give you some tools. . . . There's no rush, you're working, exercising and doing the right things. If you think there are any issues, however, let me know. I'll see you in three months. Let's get that bone scan for now."

I gave the requisition for the bone scan to Ann. She needed to make the call herself to arrange it. This gives the patient some responsibility for the resolution of his or her problem. We shook hands, and I moved on to the next case. As one of my colleagues once said to me in jest, "You gotta move product." True. Sad but real.

Three months later, Ann was back in my office. The pain was about the same. Life is busy. "I haven't had time to get the bone scan." Car pools, swim classes, overtime at work, former husband always arrives late to pick up the kids when it's his weekend . . . but life's okay—no new crises or pain setbacks. Back still hurts as before. One-foot-long patch of primarily central low back pain.

She still looked tense, guarded. *Big deal, so many people do.* Back motion was still excellent, and she noted only minimal tenderness when I applied my fingertips to the little bone tips visible under the skin, the "spinous processes," or to the muscles beside them, the paraspinals.

This was a "follow-up" visit. One half-hour instead of the initial one hour was booked. Once again, we reviewed the fact that the bone scan might tell us whether there is persisting inflammation, meaning possible movement at the "lytic" (piece of missing bone) defect that was seen on the x-ray. She said she would make the appointment for the test.

Once again, I briefly talked about the roles of stress, anxiety, and "other stuff" on pain. Muscles can excessively contract, and a dollar's worth of pain becomes 50 dollars' worth. Wounds in stressed rats seem to take longer to heal than similar wounds in nonstressed rats. The mind and the body can really interact with each other and lead to painful consequences. I left the room, saying, "Give me a call if you want me to arrange for a psychologist, social worker, or psychiatrist to help you through something. I'm not an expert in treating those issues, and those people are. Just let my secretary know, and I'll call you back." I desired more dialogue with Ann, but once again she didn't want to talk much.

A month went by and my secretary got a telephone call and provided me with the message "Ann would like to see a psychologist for the problems you discussed." I called her back. Ann indicated that there were a few things she'd like to talk about with a psychologist. I didn't ask her what they were. I was just happy she had called me. I referred her to a local psychologist with whom I'm familiar.

Two months later, Ann was back for a follow-up appointment. She couldn't afford to see a psychologist. She had gone twice to a psychiatrist—psychiatrists are medical doctors and are paid in Canada by the government medical system, but psychologists are absolutely not. She noted that her sessions had focused mainly on her early childhood. She had not returned for further counseling. She did not see the relevance.

How's your pain? "Much better." *What percentage of the pain do you think is better?* "Around 90 percent." Wow. What was going on here? What had happened to cause such a change? I was really intrigued to discover Ann's pain solution.

I asked Ann what she thought the reason was for the improvement. She answered, "Did you see him in the waiting room?" "See who?" I ask. "Well, that guy who you did not see in the waiting room *was* my boyfriend. I thought about what you said about stress and pain. He was a very difficult man. He could be very quiet, for days hardly saying a word, but on other days he was explosive and violent. During those times my kids would hide in the closet. He never hit, but he sure came close, countless times. For a while I thought I could handle him, but then I realized that he was up to no good. I was not myself around him, and neither were my children. When I finally kicked him out, 90 percent of my back pain disappeared within a few days, and it's been so much better ever since."

What had gone on here? What factors had led to Ann's fairly dramatic pain reduction? My analysis is that, yes, Ann had "real pain" coming from the defective (spondylolysis) area in her back. Maybe there was micromotion going on at the spondylolytic defect, where there normally should not be any, and this had led to the production of pain. She also likely had a second type of pain caused by tightness of muscles and ligaments, which can be caused by mood, anxiety, tension, or "stress." This second pain lessened or became much more tolerable when the "stressful boyfriend" was removed. Putting the concepts together, the spondylolysis had led to a situation whereby the muscles and ligaments surrounding the area were more susceptible to any physical or emotional stresses. Unpacking boxes and having a mood-challenged boyfriend might have led to painful surrounding musculature and much back pain.

Ann's angst associated with her boyfriend had created a cascade of emotional and thereafter physical changes, ultimately leading to painful muscles and ligaments and possibly other structures. Eliminating a stressful event, in this case, the obnoxious, controlling boyfriend, had shut down the "noxious" or painful stimuli which were hammering the back. The muscles started to unwind and heal, and the pain began to fade away. The squirting of adrenaline from the adrenal glands had eased up. An elevated heart rate might have lessened, as well.

The pain was not in Ann's mind. It was in the muscles or ligaments or other structures. Dealing with the mind by dealing with the life problem that was disturbing the mind, led to a powerful physical recovery.

After Ann "figured out" what was stressing her tissues, her pain decreased dramatically. She still experienced some pain from the spondylolysis, but it was much less and easier to control. Her newfound knowledge about what factors might have contributed to her worsening pain gave her this control.

The message for all of us is to try to "figure out" our stuff. Sometimes help from a professional such as a psychiatrist, psychologist, or social worker may be required. Sometimes not. Ann had a real, x-ray-proven problem, but the x-ray didn't explain everything. You may have a pain in your neck or back or other part of your body that could benefit from a little self-contemplation.

Read a few more stories to find out more about how life and love and the "whole damn thing" can have an impact on your pain, how others have dealt with their pain, and what journeys they went on to resolve their issues.

3

I'm So Tired of the Chronic Fatigue and Pain

A Paul Simon song keeps running through my brain and stimulates me to tell Mandy's story. Mr. Simon sings about a man being bone-tired. He's doing 900 sit-ups a day, and then he's painting his hair "the color of mud." The cryptic lyrics speak to me about how we do so many mindless, endless, and exhausting activities in our quest to be whole, fulfilled, and who knows what. We want to look young, act young, but often we aren't teenagers—and we paint our hair and ourselves into a corner and it doesn't look that good . . . like mud! Sometimes we're spinning yards and meters of pointless and colorless yarn and we don't even need the wool. We ache and we're tired and we just don't know how we got that way.

Chronic fatigue syndrome is a state of extreme fatigue that is now acknowledged to be a medical condition. Certainly it is covered by that blanket term "controversial," and some physicians may question its validity, but it is an entity that in my opinion exists and should not be belittled. As with fibromyalgia syndrome and headache and back pain and so many other medical disorders, it is necessary to get behind, in front, on top, and everywhere around the problem to truly understand and treat it. Here's a story about one woman's quest to unravel the spool of fatigue and pain that she was experiencing.

Mandy was referred to me by her family doctor. A crisp consult note was faxed. I try to review all the consults every few days to prioritize them. If it's a problem that I think needs immediate attention, I'll indicate that to my secretary. It is not always easy to establish this priority list. This case seemed pretty serious.

Mandy was noted to be a divorced woman who had not been working at her usual Armed Forces position for the past six months—the note said because of "severe fatigue." Pain was a problem, too.

I saw Mandy about a month after the consult was sent. She was a taut-looking, 37-year-old woman of medium height, with her hair pulled back with an elastic band. I told her I was a physiatrist and explained what physiatry involves. I informed her that I often ask lots of questions about people's lives and if she wasn't sure why I asked any particular one, she should tell me and I would do my best to explain. She looked a bit wary but nodded her head.

A few details about her life were needed to start the interview. Divorced for how many years? Eight. We briefly discussed how it had not been amicable. Kids? No, never had any. Living arrangements? Living in a rented bungalow. Mother had moved in recently—not a great situation. Mother's boyfriend had kicked her out of their shared townhouse. Not the first time this had happened. But this was the first time Mother had actually moved into Mandy's home. She had never really gotten along with her mother, and the atmosphere was apparently a bit tense.

Any medications currently being taken? A few Tylenol, a few Advil here and there. She had been diagnosed with pernicious anemia in the past and received a vitamin B_{12} injection once a month. This is a type of anemia (not enough blood cells swimming around in your blood) that occurs as a result of an inability to absorb an important vitamin, B_{12}, which is obtained from meat, fish, poultry, eggs, and dairy products. As long as she received the injections and her laboratory tests were in the normal range, she was fine. So, although vitamin B_{12} deficiency can be a cause of underlying fatigue and even nerve damage, or "neuropathy," this did not appear be the case with Mandy.

Asking about medications sometimes reveals a lot about the patient and not just the "what, how often, for what" type of information that a physician or pharmacist might seek. Knowing that a person is taking large amounts of over-the-counter pain medication can convey information about the person's suffering. The person is in effect stating that she is hurting and needs medication to soothe the aches. Simple. Or that she doesn't like to take "strong" medication: "I had a relative who was hooked on some addictive stuff, and I don't want to get like that." More complicated. Or she never took any kind of analgesic other than acetaminophen, aspirin, or ibuprofen. Or s/he had a doctor who refused to prescribe narcotics. Even more complicated.

If large amounts of narcotics are being ingested, other kinds of information could be interpreted. Maybe the patient (a) is in more pain than "average," whatever that is, (b) is having more trouble than usual coping with the pain, (c) had a previous addiction problem, or (d) is not having any issue at all but is just "in pain." It gets complicated because, as the patient's doctor, I certainly don't want to jump to any wrong conclusions, but at the same time I have to be constantly evaluating the medical and social circumstances and cues. A previous addict now on escalating narcotics for neck pain may need closer monitoring, and stricter limits may need to be set. And assistance from my addiction colleagues may be required.

Trouble coping with a given painful condition may mean that serious psychological and social circumstances prevail, but not necessarily so. Some pain, like that coming from injured nerves after a motorcycle trauma to the shoulder, or *plexus* (the term used to describe the bundles of nerves that run from the neck to the shoulder and arm), can be very severe: burning, shooting, and hard to cope with. I may want to obtain further social information, but if someone doesn't want to tell you about his or her past, what can be done? Not much. It's the patient who will ultimately suffer.

"What type of work do you do?" Mandy was a 10-year member of an armed forces special unit and noted that she loved her job. She explained that physical and thinking skills were required, but she couldn't go into greater detail. There didn't seem to be any deep, dark secrets lurking in the background, but obviously I could not know this for certain.

"What were the first symptoms noted, and when did they start?" This is a common question of mine to try to ascertain the chronological beginnings of the first symptoms that my patients experienced. So many times a fall or a time when pain symptoms really intensified is initially mentioned, but I usually encourage the patient to go further back in time. When did you *really* start to notice pain or fatigue? This inevitably starts the history a few years earlier. Many people tend to ignore the early periods and aspects of their illness. They shrug off a minor swelling of the abdomen (which could be a sign of uterine or abdominal cancer), chest pain that intermittently happens when they go up the stairs (heart disease, angina), a "little bit" of yellowing of the eyeballs (a blockage of the bile duct; if painless, may be due to a cancerous pancreatic or intestinal tumor). We're always hoping that any difficult problem we have will just go away. Makes sense. The well of denial can run very deep indeed.

Mandy reported that there "was a time when I was a little down, about five years ago, but it got better—I took a month or two off work and that was that. . . . I was pretty tired then. . . ." She was describing a bout of depression, so common in today's society. This was a fact I would keep in the back of my mind but its relevance was unknown. I consider depression to be a risk factor for the development of pain or fatigue. But not every risk factor leads to an illness. Not all smokers develop lung cancer. I talk about pain risk factors in Chapter 6.

So, some relevant medical events may have started five years ago. Mandy noted that two years ago she began experiencing pain in her neck and shoulder area and fatigue. Wearing her helmet would bother her; the weight of it seemed to be the issue. Her belt, which could hold a gun holster, grenades, bullets, a metal flashlight. and other paraphernalia, seemed to bother her lower back on occasion. Army and police personnel frequently have to carry a fair bit of weighty material on their trunks and backs, which takes an extra toll on their bodies. And heavy backpacks create back pain in many high school and college students.

The fatigue was associated with poor sleep and a general achiness. Mundane tasks at work and at home were simply becoming harder to do. She didn't feel she could concentrate adequately or that she had enough energy to deal with her work duties.

The frequent shift work prolonged the agony: three long 12-hour shifts, then one or two days off, nights, days, middays—a tough schedule. Shift work can disturb the usual day-to-day, or "circadian," rhythm of our lives. My patients describe how they feel displaced, woozy, and lethargic if they are changing work time shifts on a regular basis. It's hard on the body and the mind. My grandmother would say, "That can't be a good thing for you," and research seems to agree. Being aware of the issues, however, can help, and by planning more rest time, eating well and regularly, and ensuring that you are adequately hydrated, you can avoid some of shift work's problems.

Mandy's affect was kind of flat. She was pleasant but not very emotional. Maybe I was listening to the equivalent of an army report from a soldier—she answered the questions but didn't provide many details. Tentative. And why shouldn't she be? We had not yet established a trusting relationship. This is a common theme when a doctor meets a patient for the first time.

The family doctor had written that all blood tests and x-ray investigations were negative. Fatigue is such a huge symptom and can be the presenting one for hundreds of diseases and medical problems. Imagine the family doctor trying to fit the problem "I'm tired" into the 10- to 15-minute time slot that was allocated that day. Let me see: cancer, anemia, nutritional deficiency, rheumatoid arthritis, immune disease, multiple sclerosis, bowel disease, anxiety, depression, the aftermath of a viral illness—they can all initially present as "I'm just pooped," and it's the family doctor who usually has to sort things out before "the specialist" may get a crack at the case.

Fatigue is just so broad a symptom and crosses over the borderlines of so many diseases. It's heard at parties, and students talk about it endlessly. There is even now a "sleep medicine" specialty; doctors keep people holed up overnight in facilities that monitor their eyelid movements, brain waves, and leg perturbations to come up with a sleep diagnosis. Obstructive sleep apnea, a relatively new diagnosis, can cause fatigue, nighttime snoring, and choking. It is often present in thick-necked, obese individuals. Wives, husbands, boyfriends, and girlfriends report "freaking out" when they see their partner, in the middle of sleep, stop breathing for 20 to 30 seconds or more, sputter, cough, and then start to breathe again. Sleep studies help to diagnose this problem, and treatment can be offered. In my opinion, sometimes the "sleepologists" (sleep medicine experts) make too huge a deal about fatigue and insomnia, over-medicalizing the state of "being tired." People's busy lives, stresses, strains, and troubles obviously affect sleep, and attending to those concerns is, most often, the answer, rather than sending someone for an expensive test. But there is certainly a place for the new sleep technology, and many patients have been helped by the treatments provided, such as CPAP (continuous positive airway pressure), an oxygen delivery system that improves blood oxygen levels and, correspondingly, sleep.

I digress, but these are some of the issues that, as the physician, I have to think about in trying to get to the root of many problems.

Mandy didn't seem to have any particular disease that could explain her fatigue. As indicated, her vitamin B_{12} malabsorption problem had been adequately treated for years, and her B_{12} blood levels were fine. She had no joint swelling or stiffness, no unusual skin rashes or eye problems, and no heel pain (symptoms seen in immune-related diseases like "lupus," or systemic lupus erythematosus [SLE], or Reiter's syndrome). Her bowels moved, but less frequently as she was somewhat constipated. There was nothing specific!

Because of her reservedness, I just didn't know how much more to ask about her personal life—that's always a dilemma. It's her first visit. We're trying to trust each other, and I can imagine hearing, "Here is Finestone probing into the details of my personal life. Let him fix my fatigue and pain first, and then he can ask me about my feelings." I struggle with these types of issues daily. On the one hand, people have to wait two to six months to see me, there is pressure to diagnose, and therefore I want to get things done quickly. On the other hand, patients have to feel confident that the information is being provided to a trustworthy individual who will actually listen.

Also, if there is some sort of disability or insurance claim involved, I am aware that the patient is concerned that any "personal" information will be revealed to the third party (e.g., insurance company). And this is not entirely wrong. Sometimes patients' personal backgrounds (such as issues that occurred during childhood) are used against them. Their childhood events, not asked about when they applied for coverage, suddenly, according to the insurance company, become the primary reasons for their new pains, and disability benefits are therefore denied. This is cruel, but it is a commonplace event in the insurance industry.

In my opinion, that's usually the wrong type of reasoning. We enter every situation as who we are: we may be nervous, be a "worrier," have depression, or have been exposed to difficult childhood or adult life situations. That is part of who we are, and, although it is possible that these factors could affect our physical health, no one should be punished as a result. Wishful thinking. Mandy briefly alluded to her marriage to a mean, verbally abusive man. She felt that she was definitely over this relationship and never thought about him.

Her "mother situation" appeared to be another complicating issue. Mandy's parents had separated when she was young. She had never perceived her mother as supportive emotionally or financially. Now her mother had nowhere to stay, and Mandy had reluctantly taken Mom into the house.

Hmm . . . lots of information, but what do these issues have to do with fatigue, pain, or life? I didn't know yet, but the antennae were up. My medical detective radar system has noted over the years that past events such as those experienced by Mandy don't always lead nowhere. They can correlate with events later on, with headaches, abdominal pain, neck pain, and, if they drain the whole system, fatigue.

I decided to stop questioning and move on to the physical exam. Chest and heart examinations were fine. Next was the musculoskeletal part of the examination, basically the muscles, ligaments, tendons, and bones. The neck muscles were tender on the right and left, as were the trapezius muscles. But her neck moved very well. The thoracic and lumbar area muscles were tender, as well, but she didn't have tons of tender joints to fit the diagnosis of fibromyalgia (another diagnosis or symptom, which is discussed in Chapter 5). Her back moved well but ached a bit when she was leaning forward and back—no big deal.

There was no weakness, loss of feeling, or abnormalities when I tapped her knees and ankles for her reflexes. These three exams—strength, sensation, and reflex testing—make up part of the "neurological examination."

Checking the x-ray reports provided little help—no arthritis, no fractures. Blood tests were okay, B_{12} level was fine, and hemoglobin (what you look for to see if there is a low blood count, or anemia) was robust.

It was time now to shift into high gear. I had to take all these bits of information and decide what's next. Did I have enough information to make a diagnosis? Not really! There was pain. Yes, I could diagnose muscle strain or "myofascial pain," which is pain involving trapezius, parathoracic, and lumbar spinal muscles in isolation. That just didn't seem like enough, however. And I didn't think I was missing a strange medical problem, but I always have to keep that thought in the back of my mind. Sometimes it is a haunting thought. With experience and time, the fear of missing a diagnosis lessens. But it never goes away.

What was going on? Why such a deep fatigue that was actually preventing Mandy from pursuing the work she loved? The antennae, which were receiving radar waves of possible negative aftereffects of past childhood and adulthood events, were certainly up. This business about her mother might be nothing, but it didn't sound like it. I was also not getting warm and fuzzy feelings that Mandy was "in touch" with herself. She just didn't appear to relate nonphysical events to her health, not unlike about 75 percent of our society (my estimate), but I wasn't sure.

It's time to get out the pain explanation and treatment diagram (see Appendix), a one-page diagram I use both (a) to explain the nature of the patient's illness so the person can go home with something to consult later on, and (b) to try to figure out more information/clues about the patient's illness and then initiate new specific treatments. It's another path on the patient's and the physician's journey.

Together, Mandy and I went through various factors that can cause or aggravate muscle or ligament pain and fatigue. Poor or nonrefreshing sleep is noted to sometimes be a trigger for muscle pain or fatigue or to be a result of these issues. Sometimes, however, poor sleep develops a life of its own and must be "treated" as if it's a cause. I often say that we all know how we feel when we can't sleep or sleep poorly for even two or three days. We're cranky, forgetful, sometimes angry, and generally less tolerant of everything. Therefore, I told Mandy that a very small dose of a medication such as amitryptyline (an old drug called Elavil that used to be one of the most popular antidepressant drugs in the world) might help to restore her sleep cycle and make her feel slightly better overall.

I never say that Elavil is a "pain pill" even though others may say that it is, because inevitably the patient is disappointed in its ability to decrease pain. The sleep-inducing effect of Elavil is a side effect of the drug—it's not fancy, it's cheap, it's not addicting, and it works . . . by providing a slightly improved and prolonged sleep. It may cause some morning grogginess, dry eyes, dry mouth, or problems urinating, but in my experience these don't occur with small doses (5 to 30 mg taken at about 8 P.M.).

Mandy indicated that her new boss was a bit nasty. He didn't seem to understand what she was going through and kept telling her she should just go back to work "and get over it," whatever that means.

We discussed the role of exercise. People who are fatigued and in pain don't do enough exercise, and it's a bit of a challenge to get an exercise program going. "If I do too much exercise, I'll get tired, and then my problems will worsen," is what patients often say. I explained to Mandy that regular exercise increases endurance and would, therefore, help with fatigue. The exercise might not immediately improve the pain, but if she could do more, that would be an obvious health benefit.

Mandy then informed me that she got a lot of exercise riding and taking care of her five horses. The horses lived in a barn, which she rented, and each day she took them out and brushed and groomed them. Her eyes were a bit watery when she discussed the love she felt for her animals. When she rode them, it was about the only time during the day that she felt relatively "normal." The horses seemed to be able to sense and respond to her mood. They had become part of her family, and she noted that she needed to continue this mentoring relationship wherever she was.

A typical dilemma: on the one hand, she was fatigued, drained, unable to work; on the other hand, she was spending hours a day tending the barns, using a pitchfork, feeding the animals. If a video camera were trained on her it might look like she really wasn't disabled at all. The use of video cameras is quite common in today's insurance- and law-oriented society; I have frequently been sent an accompanying videocassette or DVD, arranged without the patient's knowledge, showing activities that a patient was involved with. How are the Family Doctor, the physical therapist, and I supposed to react when viewing such footage? Does the fact that bales of hay are being heaved for an hour a day mean that my patient can return to full-time work? Does it mean that the person is not sleeping 14 hours a day before and after the activity?

I have—too many times—seen colleagues rush to proclaim a particular patient a fraud or imposter after seeing such images, and I think that is wrong. Video images may leave out much information. The image producers always try to cut out any image that may actually indicate that the patient has a problem (e.g., limping, grimacing, slowing down, switching to another arm). How much videotape is left lying on the cutting room floor? We'll never know. How many codeine tablets did the patient take before the activity to avoid pain? The video cannot demonstrate that, either.

Still, seeing someone portage a canoe for three hours after he has told you he has trouble getting out of bed can be a powerful image. I have rarely seen any truly damning videos that have completely changed my opinion about a particular case, but it has happened.

Back to the patient . . . she was sleeping many hours a day. Her concentration and memory were poor, and taking care of herself and her horses was about all she could do. I had no doubts about the legitimacy of her illness. I did counsel her that perhaps taking care of one to two—instead of five—horses would make sense, but this was not advice she could follow just then. She needed her "rein" on her horses to hold onto her sanity. She was getting enough exercise; unlike the case with most of my other patients, a lack of exercise didn't seem to be part of her problem.

So, we discussed the roles of sleep (or lack of it) and exercise. Often I then talk about ergonomics, the "machine-body interface." This was not a major issue in Mandy's case (see Chapters 4 and 11, which delve to a greater extent into ergonomic issues), but I did discuss the role of heavy equipment, such as that slung from belts and carried in knapsacks, and the office environment. Lugging a heavily laden belt around can play a role in initiating low back pain.

So what came next? What else did I think was worth discussing, delving into as a means of improving, decreasing, and or even eliminating the fatigue and/or pain?

First, I usually ask my patient if she thinks there are any other conditions, issues, or events that could potentially be affecting her muscle pain. These may be issues such as diet or obesity or other factors that the patient is thinking about. We discuss them. Obesity, I usually say, is not the cause of a particular neck or back pain. It seems obvious to say that it doesn't help to be carrying around an extra sack of potatoes in your arms and that maybe the extra weight forces you to assume a certain posture . . . but too much weight rarely seems to be the *cause* of the pain problem.

"Anything else, Mandy? Anything else that you think could be aggravating your pain or causing increased fatigue, or both?" If complete silence pervades the room after this question, I usually don't stack up my papers, collect my marbles, and leave the examination room . . . but I may be a little disappointed. The patient's self-analysis and own "figuring out" are often the key to coming up with a treatment plan, but this is not always needed.

Sometimes, maybe 50 percent of the time, patients will offer a little kernel, a reflection, a suggestion: "Stress?" I will frequently ask them what they mean. "What could stress have to do with your particular pain or fatigue problem?" I am interested in how they think, what relationship between mind and body they are wondering about. I am trying to build more therapeutic bridges between the two, if appropriate.

Most commonly, the patient will say, "You know, stress makes you pull up on your shoulders, tighten your neck muscles, that kind of stuff. . . ." This is what I want to hear. The person is recognizing relationships between life and matter, between blood and guts and feelings. It can start off an exciting intricate trip down a straight or twisting road . . . or maybe not.

An explanation about the effect of stress and other life events on one's health may then follow. Of course, every case is different, but my treatment sheet has a list of things that can have a possible effect on anyone's pain or fatigue. "As you can see, Ms. Smith, this list was preprinted, not written for you."

The list of things that can worsen, aggravate, or affect pain includes (1) life in general, (2) financial problems, (3) physical abuse, (4) sexual abuse, (5) alcoholism (yours or a family member's), and (6) anger. I note that these are but a few events that, in my experience, can sometimes play a role in a person's pain or fatigue. There are also a few blank lines so that the patient can add any other relevant risk factors.

Sometimes I will note what a distant psychiatric friend called "the lower-lip quiver sign": a mild to more intense vibrating or shaking of the lower lip. He thought it was a visual response to a deep-seated issue such as a history of childhood abuse that had rarely been talked about previously. Sometimes the patient will start to cry. Sometimes there is anger: "You mean you think because I'm depressed or was abused, that that's why I'm in pain." I don't have a pat answer, but I will usually say, "I'm not saying anything. I'm here to help you. In my experience, sometimes these types of issues, problems, events could be playing some kind of role in your pain or fatigue. You tell me." We talk about how tight, contracted muscles can hurt and how further squeezing and contraction of injured muscles because of painful memories, nightmares, driving fears, or generalized anxiety can aggravate an injured body part and lead to a heightened pain experience.

Well, Mandy was still in front of me. She frankly had never thought about possible roles that feelings and the mind in general could have on her pain. She was open to the idea, however.

Together, we then started to explore some of her past issues. She was divorced and her husband had been abusive, but she really thought she had dealt with this difficult time in her life. We talked about her mother—how she had had to change roles and take care of her mother instead of the other way around. Her mother would talk to her for hours on the telephone, and Mandy would have difficulty cutting her off. Mandy's facial expression altered when we talked about this subject.

"How much is this mother issue bothering you?" I asked. "A lot. My mother was not there for my sister and me. She drank. We came home after school and had to fend for ourselves. I wish she would just leave me alone and let me be!" Now Mother had no money and no place to stay. She was living with Mandy. Tempers were flaring, stress was everywhere, and pain and fatigue were escalating.

What to do? Well, Mandy was a very receptive and gentle individual. We went back to the pain explanation and treatment diagram. In my opinion, her pain and fatigue were totally physical. This did not mean, however, that psychological, social, or emotional factors were not playing minor or major roles. Her mother seemed to be currently playing a major role in her life. I noted that I was not a psychologist but said that it seemed to me that psychological work with this and likely/possibly other issues could yield rich fruit. Psychotherapy could allow those muscles to unwind, those energy gates to open. Along with physical therapy, increased exercise, and less horse work, it could help Mandy to actually improve and get better.

"Could I go back to work, Dr. Finestone?" "Eventually, why not?" I indicated. I thought improvement was possible. "How do I do all this, Dr. Finestone?" "Let's start off with a psychologist," I said. The Armed Forces had one available as part of their health service to their employees. Also, I asked Mandy to start writing about what she had gone through, as a child and more recently. "Be detailed, and just let it all hang out." I sometimes call this "literary therapy." It allows my patients to explore areas where they had previously never been.

Mandy was a model patient. She immediately found a psychologist. The psychologist sounded like a very practical individual who immediately recognized the deleterious role of Mandy's mother. Strict rules were placed on the length of telephone conversations and encounters with Mother. Mandy's mother was informed that she couldn't speak to her daughter more than once a day—this was a reduction from the usual 20 times per day!

Mandy started to swim. She wrote in her journal daily. I saw her every three months. She needed pain medication for her shoulder and neck area pain, but less often. Her sleep slowly became less troublesome.

The story does have a happy but not perfect ending. After one and a half years of being on disability, Mandy decided to return to work—a bit shaky, a bit worried, and still fatigued—but she felt ready to return, and fortunately she had a very supportive boss who was willing to accept her still-present disabilities. She started out working mainly in the office and slowly moved out into the field. I encouraged her at every visit, as there was a lot to encourage her about. She was more animated and more in control of her destiny than before. A specific return-to-work schedule was devised, and the family doctor and I both signed it. The plan called for slow increases in time at work, beginning with two half-days per week. There were a few false starts, but over five months Mandy eventually returned to full-time work.

On her last visit, I asked her which part of her treatment was most helpful to her. What had she learned most about during the past months? "Dr. Finestone, I learned how my feelings affect me, my muscles, and my energy levels. You, my family doctor, and my psychologist taught this to me. Thanks!" *What could be a more rewarding case?* I thought to myself. She and I had learned much in our journey together. Some pain detective work had helped to reestablish buried physical and emotional connections, and the patient and many parts of society had helped with the rest.

Many society related pieces had to be sewn together to make this pain and fatigue garment a successful fit—a family doctor, a specialist, a supportive workplace, a kind and competent psychologist, a decent disability plan that paid Mandy during her work absence, and an innate intelligence and a willingness to think in a way that was different for her. Maybe the fact that she didn't have any children and could concentrate on her personal healing made a difference, as well. It takes time and a focused effort to heal, and we can't always find that special zone, even when we feel ready to do so.

Mandy presented to her physician with symptoms of pain and fatigue, symptoms that are common, even omnipresent in today's society. Careful listening to both rule in and rule out many medical illnesses was required. Physical examination of multiple body parts and imaging and blood tests were also required as part of the diagnostic process. The pain and the fatigue were physically based, but the role of the mind and the effect of current and past social and psychological influences on the mind certainly influenced the body. Mandy's case cannot be expected to explain every person's chronic fatigue state. But many of Mandy's issues are universal and worth considering in other similar scenarios.

Chronic worry and anxiety are fatiguing. And chronic worry and anxiety affect our immune system, our musculoskeletal system, our neurological system, our digestive system, our hearts, the way we clench our teeth . . . the effects are vast and sometimes seem overwhelming. Mandy was dealing with a dependent parent who hadn't been emotionally available to Mandy when Mandy was young. Mandy unfortunately had become immersed in a difficult marital relationship, from which she had extricated herself quite nicely. Her job was a physically and emotionally demanding one, and eventually her body simply couldn't handle the load. Her horses helped to calm her spirit, but the physical demands of caring for them were often too much. That's what happens, and similar scenarios will continue to happen as long as human beings roam this earth and as-yet unexplored universes.

Chronic fatigue syndrome with or without pain is a fact. But people read the same information and interpret it differently. Unfortunately, that's a fact, too. Mandy listened to others, to her body, and to her inner self. It took time and effort, from multiple directions, for her to heal. But heal she did, and I hope she is still on her healing path. Because the healing never stops.

4

ELBOW GREASE

The activities we perform with our arms, legs, backs, necks, and minds often determine our futures and fortunes. Sometimes it is the very specific tasks or goals we take on that predict that a particular pain syndrome will occur, and on other occasions it is a complex set of circumstances. I like my patients to be vigilant about their personal body actions and how they relate to their symptoms, but not obsessively so. It is a fine line.

Judy was a 47-year-old woman employed as an office cleaner. Her family doctor referred her to me because of "unremitting right elbow pain." Chances are that if a specialist like me is evaluating a particular medical problem, then the complexity has ratcheted up a bit. Family doctors can handle the majority of musculoskeletal problems. Many to most of the problems relating to our muscles and ligaments eventually sputter and burn out without our even needing a visit to the doctor. That sore back after gardening, the tender ankle after a basketball game, the neck aggravation after sitting hunched over a three-hour exam, the burning forearm and hand after too many hours doing crafts with the glue gun . . . these nagging annoyances do usually go away, dissipating into the humors of time within days to months—that is, assuming, of course, that we can stop doing the particular activity that led to the problem in the first place. Sports medicine, a discipline that often looks after sport- and work-related musculoskeletal problems, is certainly a needed medical discipline. Sometimes we doctors do poke fun at it, however, by saying that "sports medicine is the medicine practiced whereby you do as much therapy and as many interventions as you can before the problem gets better on its own!" Facetious, yes, but it rings the bell of truth for many practitioners.

Judy's pain had not gone away and had been going on for eight months. She worked Monday to Friday in a large office complex, mopping, cleaning, polishing floors, and dusting. "What was the pain, when did it start and under what circumstances was it happening?" I asked her. The pain started off as a mild ache over the outer part of her elbow. At first it was noticed mostly on Thursday afternoons. By Friday the outer elbow would hurt even more, but usually after a weekend's rest she'd improve. On Monday she'd usually be fine.

Slowly but surely, the pain began to start earlier on in the week—Wednesday, then Tuesday, then Monday, until a weekend's rest didn't help much at all.

Now the pain was constant and gnawing, and when she gripped the broom, the vacuum cleaner handle, or even a doorknob, pain would shoot up the back of her hand and land at her elbow. Holding onto her car's steering wheel aggravated the situation, as well. She could carry shopping bags only if they were filled with the lightest of articles, because, otherwise, gripping the bag handles was just too painful.

Judy was still working, in pain, but only because she really needed the money. Her husband had recently been diagnosed with prostate cancer. He was waiting to be operated on and in the meantime was not working. The construction company he worked for was small, and therefore he was not receiving any disability or health benefits. Money was tight.

Judy's boss was being very kind, and fellow workers were helping her out on the heavier tasks, such as mopping and moving furniture. This is what happens to employees who are well liked and respected at work. Fellow employees go to bat for the respected worker, and he or she somehow holds on to the job. If the employee is not liked, "forget about it." Judy felt really good about her work situation but somewhat guilty about imposing greater responsibilities on her cleaning coworkers.

A systematic approach is vitally important in the practice of medicine. There is so much to remember. Doctors needs to group information into categories, and they need to remember multiple systematic approaches to asking questions, performing a physical exam, and ordering specific tests. I started off with the "PQRSTU" method of pain description, **p**ain, its **q**uality, **r**adiation, **s**everity and **t**iming, and **u**nder what circumstances it occurs.

Judy's pain was achy, sore, and sometimes burning. She said that it radiated (a fancy term doctors use to mean moving from one place to another) from her elbow down into the back of her hand. (I can often tell whether the patient has been to many, too many, therapists and/or doctors by whether she uses the term "radiate" during the course of my interview.) There was no tingling or numbness, symptoms that one often experiences if suffering from an injured nerve in the arm or neck. Judy said that the pain was fairly focused in one area of the side of her elbow, which one sees in a muscle, ligament, or bone problem. It wasn't excruciating, but it was "very painful." There were no associated facial rashes or skin changes, which one can see with inflammation-related diseases like systemic lupus erythematosus (SLE), more commonly referred to as "lupus." Pain was not worse at night, which can occur when a bone tumor is present. In medicine, "pertinent negatives"—symptoms the patient does *not* have—can be just as important as positive findings. I want to know what the patient is not experiencing just as much as what she is. Missing a diagnosis may have greater repercussions than finding out the right one. Emergency department physicians may not care much what the cause of their patients' chest pain is, but they need to ensure that an untreated heart attack is not walking out of the hospital doors.

It sounded like "tennis elbow" could be the problem. I'll describe what this is in greater detail later on, but for now let's say it is a problem of the tendon entering the elbow bone. Medical students are told that 90 percent of patients' diagnoses should be obtained after the "history," the patient's story. This is so true. The physical exam is said to give you another 5 percent of the diagnostic information, and 5 percent more comes from blood tests, x-rays, and other tests.

Of course, it's not always like that. Sometimes a particular blood or imaging test can hit a home run, such as an MRI (magnetic resonance imaging) that shows the presence of a ligament-based cancerous tumor when all other tests are normal. That happened to me once, when examining the elbow area of an 18-year-old woman. She was experiencing right elbow pain and mild tenderness over the back of her elbow. When she brushed her arm lightly against her school locker, the elbow felt uncomfortable. But all tests were normal. That is, the x-ray and the bone scan were normal. I decided to order an MRI because I felt that I needed more information. This was not a pain due to stress, as so many medical and allied health professionals before me had indicated. The surprising results of the MRI came back. The woman had a sarcoma (cancer) of the triceps tendon, which was successfully surgically removed. This type of case can happen, but of course it is not common. It points out that the consequences of not recognizing a particular disease are more daunting than an accountant's missing a line on a financial statement. This weighs a bit heavily on my mind sometimes, but obviously I cannot be too worried about missing a diagnosis or I'll never rely on my judgment and I'll be ordering MRIs for every patient. That would not be good medicine. It would be the medicine of fear.

In Judy's case, I needed more information. I examined her, that is, I performed the "physical examination" part of most doctors' repertoires. We're supposed to examine the "joint above and the joint below" the problem area. That's to rule out "referred pain," pain coming from another source. Because Judy's problem was around her elbow, her neck and wrist/hand therefore had to be checked. Her neck motion was fine and painfree. The muscles around the neck, the trapezeii (those bulky muscles at the top of our shoulders, between the neck and the tip of the shoulder), the cervical extensors (back of neck), and those around the shoulder blade (rhomboids, levator scapulae) were not tender when I dug my fingertips into them. I quickly moved to the elbow region.

I palpated, or pressed, the outer elbow, pushing downward from the skin toward the bone below it. When I am practicing this part of the physical examination, I try to visualize all of the structures that my fingers are pressing on. This not only makes my medical life more thoughtful and interesting but also allows me to be more vigorous about the source of the person's pain. Skin, then fat, then tendon, then bone. The medical texts tell us that the tendon, the tough leather-like band that comes off the muscle, transforms itself as it is heading toward its "home," the bone of the elbow. So muscles become tendons and tendons soon transform into a substance called fibrocartilage. The fibrocartilage, further down the line, calcifies (takes on calcium and hardens) and become what are called "Sharpey's fibers." There is no clear demarcating point where this bone anchoring happens.

I sometimes explain to my patients how the attachment of tendon to bone is quite a miraculous achievement. We discuss how if we look around the room, on our clothing, in our cars, on cabinets and machines, we'll see that parts and objects are often attached to each other—metal to metal, zipper to cloth, wood to brick, paper to paper. When these attachments occur, there's always something binding the two parts: a nail, a screw, solder, glue. The "miracle" of tendon-to-bone attachments is that you don't see an attachment part. It is seamless. Through some miracle of transformation and adhesion, the tendon merges imperceptibly into the bone. When the design is still intact and whole, the tendon therefore just glides into the bone, no strings attached. The tendon escapes into a mysterious channel in the bone's surface and suddenly disappears. That's when everything is going well. It's a beautiful streamlined process, pearly and glistening but tough and unyielding.

Sometimes I go even further and ask my patients if they keep any muscles or tendons in their house. "Does any one room in your house hold more of this material than others?" Funny question maybe, but I've come to realize that health professionals probably take too much of the information they share for granted. Many people don't usually know what muscles and tendons are or do, and why should they? Maybe it's gruesome, but I point out that the meat we eat is muscle. I ask my patients to think about how the meat of a rib steak passes smoothly into the bony part. No strings, tacks, or adhesives there, just a smooth transition from the red meat into the bone. Some are shocked to hear that steak, tenderloin, chuck, London broil, flank steak, and filet mignon are actually different muscles from different parts of the cow's body. I have affixed large pictures of the muscles of the human body on the walls of my examination room. People really appreciate this, and sometimes these diagrams are their first look at the muscles and ligaments of the body.

When I palpated the back of Judy's wrist, it was tender, but only over part of the wrist, just "proximal" (doctor speak for closer to the core of the body) to the pinkie and ring fingers. Hmm. I put that information somewhere in my brain and moved on to the elbow, where most of the pain was occurring. Still, a few red lights and soft-sounding buzzers were now pulsating deep in the recesses of my gray matter, cells that are part of the brain. Why was that part of the wrist, just the outside back of the wrist, just over the two outer fingers, tender? This area usually wasn't tender to my touch in a "typical" case of tennis elbow. I would have to come back to that potentially useless or possibly precious piece of information later.

Look, feel, move. This is the mantra of the examining doctor who is practicing musculoskeletal medicine, the medicine of bones, joints, ligaments and muscles, the "flesh" of our bodies. When I had looked at Judy's elbow, there was not much to see. No redness or swelling (signs of infection or inflammation) was evident. Exquisite tenderness was noted over a quarter-size area over the outside (doctor speak: "lateral") of her elbow. She was also tender further along the forearm (doctor speak: "distal," meaning farther away from the core of the body) and, as indicated, over the back of the hand, wrist, and ring and pinkie fingers. I was mentally reviewing and repeating the physical examination results in my brain.

Her elbow and wrist joints moved well without pain. I asked her to keep her wrist cocked upward toward the ceiling while I held on to the back of her hand (to test "resisted" range of motion). She felt intense pain over the lateral elbow, the point of her previously noted tenderness. This is known as a "special" or "provocative" test.

Well, the plot was thickening. Judy experienced lateral elbow pain. There was no obvious joint or arthritic pain, and she felt elbow pain when she "pushed" her arm or gripped objects or when wrist movement was resisted. This was the pattern of a muscle-tendon or ligament problem. That is, the painful part was tender to touch, and when I stressed it by resisting movement, it hurt.

The well-known entity "tennis elbow" again, this time more boldly, marched into my mind. The doctors' term for tennis elbow is "lateral epicondylitis." The epicondyle is the bony part above the elbow, belonging to the upper arm bone, the humerus.

Tennis elbow is a few things. It can be an inflammation or swelling and redness of the attachment of a forearm tendon into the bone. Ian Goldie, a scientist in Sweden, looked at a bunch of cadaver arms and found that there were actually signs of "microtrauma," small tears and granulation tissue (spongy, early healing tissue), in the arms of people who had experienced tennis elbow. The wearing-and-tearing part seemed to be more important than actual inflammation, which is less prominent.

I remembered all of the other terms used over many years to describe "tennis elbow"—"politician's paw" because politicians have to shake so many hands, "tomato picker's blight" because of the repetitive use of the arm and especially the elbow by vegetable pickers. Lots of names for a similar problem. Most people who develop tennis elbow don't play tennis at all, but I guess the name is more attractive than "ditch digger's elbow" or "plumber's elbow" (I made these terms up, but they make sense).

But what was Judy's activity? Was there one? She was an office cleaner. I understood why her elbow could be painful, but why the back of the wrist over just the pinkie and ringer fingers? What kind of elbow grease was she applying to her cleaning tools?

Judy couldn't think of anything specific that she was doing with her right arm. "I clean," she said. "What do you clean?" I asked. "Everything. Even though it's an office, I have to clean furniture, bathtubs, walls, carpets. . . ." "You must be using some kind of tool or doing something particular, Judy. What is it? What do you hold in your hand?" "A spray bottle," she said. "Which fingers do you use?" "My pinkie and ring fingers."

The penny dropped (in today's vending machines, maybe $2.95 was deposited). Judy was spending a large chunk of the day cleaning offices and bathrooms. She pumped that spray bottle hundreds, thousands of times, spurting cleaning fluid everywhere. She "overused" her arm and developed a tenderness over her arm and wrist. She had not tennis but "spray bottle" epicondylitis.

Judy and I discussed treatment. My approach to tennis elbow has evolved over the years. I injected her elbow with a cortisone solution. This is an accepted form of treatment, but often it doesn't work or the improvement just doesn't last. In general, "tennis elbow" is not felt to be an inflammatory problem. Often there is some inflammation present, but most of the time there is, as Goldie described, tear/re-tear, that is, the tendons attached to the bone fray, heal to form a weak scar, and tear again when some type of gripping occurs, so the cycle of pain, scarring, and, likely a little inflammation continues. The injection provided Judy with good initial relief, but the relief lasted only a few weeks.

I'm going to recount another tennis elbow story now, to allow a nice transition into treatment issues for this nonlife-threatening but frequently distressing disorder. A family doctor and friend came to me with a three-year history of lateral elbow pain that had started when he hiked a few kilometers uphill, in the snow, while tightly gripping his alpine skis. Injections, physiotherapy, and tight tennis elbow "bands" around the arm just hadn't helped. Many people try the tennis elbow brace, which, via a Velcro attachment, wraps tightly around the fleshy part of the elbow below the bonier part above where the tendon enters the bone. It's worth trying but helps only some patients. And it shouldn't be used all day as the muscle beneath it will actually shrink and weaken if the brace is worn too long. He had to quit his beloved game of squash because "it was just too damn painful."

I had heard about a treatment used by a well-known physiatrist in the United States, Dr. Ernest Johnson, but I wasn't totally sure what it entailed. I called Dr. Johnson, and he was happy to send me the treatment protocol. He had never actually written a full scientific article on the subject but noted that he had described and prescribed the treatment many times. It involved the use of increasing free weights to stress the injured tissues and eventually cause a denser, painfree scar.

The treatment seemed to make some sense. The lateral elbow purportedly hurts because of tearing and incomplete healing of the tendon entry into the bone. We teach that it occurs due to overuse, that is, too much strain on the area. So I was now going to prescribe a progressive weight-training program that stresses the painful and injured tennis elbow tendons so that healing will occur? "Does that make sense?" I wondered. But apparently the treatment, by strengthening the extensor tendons attached to the elbow in a controlled, organized manner, allows healing to occur. Healing tissue called collagen is laid down in a stronger, more efficient way, and less pain results. That was the theory.

The family physician started the weight-training exercises. They were very painful to perform, and his family recounted how moaning sounds could be heard throughout the house while he slowly lowered the weight down and lifted it up. Within a month, however, he began to note significant improvement in symptoms, and in two months he was painfree. I was very excited to witness this success and have been prescribing further iterations of the exercise program ever since.

Judy started to take more breaks, used the spray bottle in her right and left hands, and began squeezing the trigger of the bottle with her index and middle fingers. These adjustments all made a huge difference. She also took up the treatment program, and, even though she was improving thanks to her new spraying techniques, the treatment seemed to really help her. I wrote about "spray bottle epicondylitis" in the journal *Canadian Family Physician*.[1] The critical message was that knowledge of the diagnosis was not enough. Diagnosing the underlying pain-causing mechanism was critical to solving patients' elbow pain. The tools we use in today's society are always changing and constantly create new environments for injury. For example, "gaming thumb" refers to injuries sustained while aggressively overusing the thumb while playing computer and other electronic-based games. The list goes on.

The novel exercise treatment I prescribed for the family physician was published several years later in *Canadian Family Physician*.[2] While others had published similar treatments, this treatment was the only "home-based" one, not requiring any specific equipment or gadgetry. I have been very gratified by the attention this article has received. A number of physicians and patients have used the treatment described, and some have told me that it has tremendously benefited them.

This chapter illustrates that not *every* musculoskeletal problem is in the "mind-body" category. But the aching symptoms do still tell many stories. And what we do with our bodies must often be closely connected to the symptoms and illnesses we experience.

Too many times, we talk about our pains as if they are divorced from anything we do with our minds or our bodies. Surely there are illnesses like pancreatic cancer where we can't always connect the dots between a certain toxic exposure, be it environmental or drug or lifestyle related, and the development of the medical problem. But that doesn't mean it's not worth considering mind-body, environment-body, and activity-body interactions. Knowledge is power in these situations because if you can figure out a new "health relationship"—I just made up that term—then the treatment possibilities can increase dramatically. Judy recognized that a specific work tool was responsible for much of her sore elbow and wrist. Changing the working environment made a huge difference. Switching arms and changing which fingers she used to press on the spray bottle trigger took pressure off those hard-working tendons. The tendons became less injured and were given the opportunity to heal. After all, healing naturally, without special potions, pills, or manipulations, is usually the best way to go on the road to recovery.

We also learn from Judy and my family doctor friend that effective treatments may come from many ideas and places. Doctors and patients must keep an open mind about what is the optimal treatment for a given disease. Knowing about the tennis elbow treatment that I first learned about from my American colleague has helped my patients with tennis elbow and also those with tendon problems in other parts of the body. There may be many other treatments offered by all kinds of practitioners. But they have to make some kind of sense, and you have to feel comfortable when they are applied. If you don't feel right about a particular type of treatment, don't do it. Make sense of your treatment, and discuss it with your provider so you can then make an informed decision about its application.

Shopping, shaking hands, picking tomatoes, playing tennis, doing plumbing, hammering nails—all can lead to a form of Judy's problem of lateral epicondylitis. Discovering the mechanism of injury and devising innovative work and home modifications can make big differences in the way the problem works out.

NOTES

1. H. M. Finestone and S. Helfenstein, "Spray Bottle Epicondylitis. Diagnosing and Treating Workers in Pain," *Canadian Family Physician* 40 (1994): 336–337.

2. H. M. Finestone and D. L. Rabinovitch, "Tennis Elbow No More: Practical Eccentric and Concentric Exercises to Heal the Pain," *Canadian Family Physician* 54 (2008): 1115–1116.

5

TEARS AND FIBROMYALGIA SYNDROME

A few years back I started an article on fibromyalgia with a brief story about Ms. Smith and Dr. Jones. It was a tale rather than an actual medical experience, but it reflected many of my thoughts about this much-maligned and misunderstood syndrome. I recount this story here and discuss some of fibromyalgia's challenging clinical features. I then share some encounters with past patients to help the reader understand fibromyalgia's differing presentations and treatments.

Fibromyalgia syndrome (FMS) is being diagnosed in hundreds of thousands of people. What is it? It is a condition involving diffuse pain, sleep disturbances, tender body points, and numerous other health problems that I discuss later on in this chapter. It desperately needs to be better understood in society today. Many health practitioners believe that it clearly exists (many also debate it), but it would help to be more aware of how and when it presents and what can be done about it. This chapter is one attempt to achieve these goals.

Fibromyalgia sufferers, in my opinion, can improve their health status. Being diagnosed with FMS does not mean one is guaranteed to be the victim of a medical condition that is filled with unending despair. So much information is available in the lay and research literature, but it is still difficult to come up with conclusive, truly helpful, meaningful material. That does not mean, however, that fibromyalgia cannot be treated in a caring and thorough manner. There are many lights at the end of the fibromyalgia tunnel, but we need to know which switches to flip and which parts need replacing in order for the bulbs to resume burning. Now let's hear that tale. . . .

Ms. Smith visited her family doctor's office in tears, crying her eyes out. Her face was flushed, her eyes were rheumy, her nose was scarlet, and the tissues she tightly clutched were a messy pulp of pink and yellow. She was ushered from the waiting room into one of the four examination rooms. The dates on the magazines indicated that they were about three years old, not too bad for a doctor's office.

Dr. Jones was an efficient young family physician. He wanted to solve this crying problem quickly, efficiently, and in a cost-effective manner.

Dr. Jones marched into the examining room and listened to Ms. Smith's chest and heart and gazed through a lighted instrument up her nose. When her pupils were subjected to a quick shot of a harsh light, they constricted quickly and with authority. They were not the pupils of a person with syphilis, which can "accommodate but not react" (e.g., constrict with reading but not to a flash of light). Time was of the essence. There were 13 people in the waiting room, and it was 4 P.M. "Ms. Smith, you are experiencing lacrimation, also known as tearing or crying. It's not a serious condition. Tears, a salty or saline solution, are produced by small lacrimal glands located on top of your eyes. The tears waft across your eyes and are collected in little bony channels called nasolacrimal ducts, then land up in your nose. That's why you often have to blow your nose when you are crying."

"I'll tell you what I want you to do." Dr. Jones reached into his medicine cupboard, which was filled with all kinds of products provided to him by visiting drug detail persons or pharmaceutical representatives. "Take this special type of medical glue and tap a few drops around your glands every three hours. The lacrimal glands will then stop producing tears, and you will stop crying. Problem solved."

Now, we know that (1) Dr. Jones is a fictional character, (2) he never actually gave Ms. Smith that speech, (3) no doctor would seriously sermonize the way Dr. Jones did, and (4) there is no such thing as lacrimal glue, although medicinal glue is used by physicians to repair skin lacerations.

A usually caring Dr. Jones would have started with the history part of the clinical examination. He would have commenced by asking Ms. Smith a few questions, such as "Why are you crying, Ms. Smith? Has anything sad or painful happened? Did you fall? Are you hurt? Did anyone die? Are you bleeding? Did anyone try to attack you?"

That is, Dr. Jones would have tried to find out why Ms. Smith was crying. Was she happy or sad? Maybe she had won a lottery. Maybe a parent had just died. Or onions were in the room. Or she had just been diagnosed with cancer. Sometimes we cry from joy, but not anywhere near as often as from sadness. You get the drift—crying can come from many sources; it can spring from many wells.

But what does this tale have to do with FMS? What is the connection between tears and fibromyalgia? Lacrimation or tearing or crying, all synonyms, is a complex human body reaction. Multiple features of the body's biochemical, neurological, physiological, anatomical, and psychological systems may come into play to produce those briny, slippery tears. Countless hankies and tissues have been laundered and thrown out, respectively, because of crying encounters and the shedding of tears at movies, gravesides, chemical plants, courts of law, emergency departments, and weddings.

How does crying start? First, there has to be some kind of stimulus. It may be emotional (like a happy or sad event), painful (like a fall, cut, or fracture), environmental (like a cold, windy, intolerable landscape) or irritating (like a sudden gust of sand or onion fumes in the eyes). The brain seems to take over at some point, producing specific stimuli, electrical impulses that project to other neural pathways, and somehow these impulses land up in those lacrimal glands, which then start pumping out the tears. And, voilà, we cry. Prolactin, a tranquilizing hormone produced by a part of the brain called the pituitary gland, may be released into the tears of sorrow but not into the tears of simple irritation. Makes sense; in times of sadness we would appreciate being soothed, and secreting prolactin may help do this.[1]

So, multiple factors, etiologies, and stimuli, coming from a gazillion emotional, physical, and environmental places, may elicit the same fairly stereotypical reaction that we call tearing or lacrimation. A mundane, seemingly simple process is not that simple after all.

And—finally we have arrived at our destination—FMS has features that make it easily comparable to tearing. FMS is a painful, diffuse affliction of the musculoskeletal system that is real and has many scientific theories behind it. Microscopic muscle changes have been reported in scientific journals. Blood flow to exercising FMS patients' muscles has been described as reduced compared to that in "normals." Cerebrospinal fluid, the crystal-clear fluid that bathes our brain and spinal cord, may contain different amounts of neurotransmitters, the stuff that helps relay information from one part of the central nervous system to another. But, like lacrimation, there may be multiple factors that can aggravate FMS and outright cause it. A physical event like crying can be triggered by a nonphysical or emotional event. Physical FMS events like the reduced blood flow and the neurotransmitter changes may happen for various sociological and psychological reasons.

In talks on the subject I often go on to say that sometimes we doctors use the "glue the ducts" approach to treating FMS. We prescribe a little exercise and a few pills. We provide a pat on the shoulder, and little thought or emotion accompanies our advice to "carry on." Instead of examining the big picture, we often focus too exclusively on the pain, like Dr. Jones and his narrow focus on the tearing and little else. We ignore the environmental, physical, psychological, and sociological circumstances that may or may not be engulfing the patient with pain due to fibromyalgia. If we focus on these issues, there is a much better chance of getting to the core of the FMS problem, where often the healing can begin. Then we can offer constructive help, effective programs, and written material that resonates in the mind of the patient.

I'm getting a little ahead of myself. Let's look at a few clinical cases that illustrate some of these issues. Then we can perhaps appreciate what it's really like to be experiencing the symptoms of FMS, the frequent suffering that accompanies it, the doctor-patient interaction, and the attempts to resolve some of its dilemmas.

BETTY

Betty, a 56-year-old married woman, was referred to me for foot pain. The balls of her feet ached, and her family doctor wondered whether shoe inserts or orthoses (actually the correct medical term, rather than the more commonly used "orthotics") would help her. (A medical term for pain in the balls of your feet is "metatarsalgia." The metatarsals are the longish bones in your feet. Any medical term that ends in "-algia" means pain involving that part and that the pain comes from something like excessive use or wear and tear rather, than inflammation.)

I happened to have her hospital chart, and I was flipping through it. About three years earlier, Betty had been seeing one of my colleagues in rheumatology, the medical specialty that focuses on the body's joints—the hinges and connections that link bone to bone all over our bodies. There are many types of joints: ball and socket, joints with specialized discs, fibrous joints, joints that move more freely, like the shoulder, and other, stiffer ones, like the attachment of the collar bone to the breast plate, or sternum.

Rheumatologists used to specialize in rheumatic diseases (ones that were joint related), such as rheumatoid arthritis and ankylosing spondylitis, and prescribed various medications to control inflammation. Some of the new rheumatological drugs are producing outstanding results, greatly decreasing joint inflammation and thus improving patients' overall function. Rheumatologists are currently the medical specialists who more frequently diagnose and treat FMS, usually after they have been consulted by the patient's family doctor or internist. Physiatrists and other pain specialists are frequently asked to assess the patient with FMS, as well.

But it was Sir William Gowers, an English neurologist and pediatrician, who coined the term "fibrositis" in 1904, describing a diffusely painful condition of the muscles rather than the joints. "Muscular rheumatism" (a term indicating that the pain was coming from the muscles and not the joints) and "lumbago" (a general term for low back pain) were lumped together under the "fibrositis" banner. Fibrositis ends with the letters "-itis," meaning inflammation. Since the painful symptoms were not felt to be caused by an inflammatory process, the term was changed to fibromyalgia in 1976. Rheumatologists from the American College of Rheumatology established criteria for its diagnosis that are used worldwide.

I find it interesting that, although rheumatologists were involved in the "creation" of FMS, so many choose to abandon it and question its existence. Like many doctors, including me, they are uncomfortable with the diagnosis and its meaning to both the doctor and the patient. Sometimes rheumatologists, and other physicians, too, seem to want to distance themselves as far as possible from fibromyalgia. Sometimes they seem to have disdain for the diagnosis, as though it were a malady reserved for emotionally weak people. The inventors are destroying their invention. That's strange, sad, and a wrong action to take.

Betty had been diagnosed with fibromyalgia, and I asked her how this condition was treating her. She replied, "Oh, I don't really have that anymore, maybe just a little." I was somewhat stunned and asked her what had happened.

"I was working as office manager of a small business that sold pool chemicals. Hiring and firing employees, payroll—it was so stressful. I felt the whole weight of the world on my shoulders. I started to experience neck pain and back pain, I slept poorly, I was tearful, and soon I was experiencing total body pain. My work performance was suffering, too."

"Well, what did you do to get better"? I asked.

"Oh, I just couldn't take it any longer, so I went to my boss and said, 'I'm not working as the manager anymore.' I told him, 'I'm coming in three days a week as a regular employee, no Saturdays or Sundays, and that's that.'"

"What happened then?"

"Well, I was a very good employee, and he agreed to my terms. My pain didn't immediately go away, but slowly and surely my neck and back pain got so much better and my sleep improved. Now I still feel achy on days when I'm tired or cold, but it's nothing like it used to be! I am also not nearly as weepy as I was."

What was going on? The controversial, often-described "chronic, untreatable, of no etiology" FMS had gotten better? The weak-kneed, stressed-out patient with FMS had actually improved? Yes, *gotten better,* and yes, *actually improved,* were the respective answers to these questions.

Is fibromyalgia really that hard to understand? Even the biblical character Job, when tested by God, felt achy and sore all over when subjected to very rigorous demands: "The night racks my bones, and the pain that gnaws me knows no rest," he laments (Job 30:17). It's easy to imagine that Job felt stressed and distraught. Some patients have described FMS as a "whole body migraine," a kind of neat, though depressing, description that may reflect some particularly difficult FMS cases.

Why all this argument about its existence, its possibility, its place in life? Why do I get asked, "Dr. Finestone, do you believe in FMS?" as if it were an unusual religion or a ritual practiced by people from another world? No one asks me if migraines or tinnitus (ringing in the ears) exist. So why FMS?

Well, let's define it. FMS is a condition in which diffuse aching and soreness are experienced, by women far more than men, in parts of the body that are both above and below the waist. To fulfill the American College of Rheumatology criteria, an individual must have at least 11 of a possible 18 fibromyalgic tender points. In addition, fatigue, headaches, poor sleep, gastrointestinal symptoms, feelings of being cold, and the feeling that one's head is not thinking properly (also called "fibro fog" by some of my patients) constitute other components of FMS. These are the symptoms and signs that a person with FMS may experience. Patients may report some of them or all of them, some of the time or all of the time. Some people may able to work and attend to most of their life necessities, and some may not. The range of suffering and disability can be vast, varying from extremely modest to severe.

Pain all over, or diffuse widespread pain, is fairly easily understood. Everyone has felt at one time or another severe aching and soreness all over, during a cold or case of influenza, when stressed, or after participation in a new sport or work activity. The presence of the tender points is not, however, the easiest concept to understand. The tender points of FMS are 18 specific predefined areas, nine on either side of the body on the body, above and below the waist. One by one, the doctor presses each area, and if the patient experiences pain, this is considered a fibromyalgic tender point. The tender points are not magical points, however. They don't mean that the person is not capable of experiencing any other tender areas on his or her body. They are points agreed on by a group of doctors who tried to study the condition systematically. However, doctors examine these fibromyalgic tender points in different ways. It can be quite confusing for the patient. According to the definition of FMS, 4 kg of pressure is supposed to be applied to each tender point. I mainly apply pressure with my thumb until the nail bed blanches.

The fibromyalgic tender points are supposed to be unusually tender and to react in a painful way when pressed on. But how is painful tenderness defined? Reacting by jumping high enough to reach the room's light fixture? Whimpering minimally when thumb pressure is applied? Uttering, "Yes, it hurts more than usual"?

I try to initially find a nontender area of the person's body. I'll press the midpoint of the front of the patient's thigh and say, "This should not be painful, but tell me if it is." If the patient finds it painful, I'll keep pressing, moving from place to place until I find a nonpainful spot. Then I press the 18 FMS tender points and for each one ask, "Does this hurt?" I ask my patients to compare the sensation to what they felt at the previously pressed nonpainful area. This all takes time, but at least there is some kind of standardization.

While some doctors consider a point as positive for tenderness only if the person jumps off the table, I mainly want to know if the area with my applied pressure hurts. Others use an algodynometer, a cylindrical metal device that looks like a bicycle pump, to supposedly deliver a standard amount of pressure (4 kg) over the tender point. It sounds good, but it doesn't frequently work, and that's why few doctors use them. The device is not really necessary, in my opinion.

The number of tender points on a given day can vary. Why shouldn't it? The tender points are specific. They are "real." But some days a person can feel achier than other days and have fewer than 11 tender points; that does *not* mean the person doesn't have FMS. Life changes, diseases vary in severity and intensity, and FMS can express itself differently on different days. That does not mean it doesn't exist.

So you have 11 or more FMS tender points, your sleep is "the pits," and you are achy all over. You're in my office, and I'm trying to approach this problem in a systematic way. I can't just jump right into the FMS diagnosis. I have to make sure that no other grave diseases are lurking in the background. As serious, important, and treatable as FMS is, it is still a "diagnosis of exclusion." That means that I must rule out other diseases such as anemia, cancer, rheumatoid arthritis, depression (which certainly can accompany FMS), hypothyroidism, and so many other possible ailments. That's not too hard. A thorough history, a complete physical exam, and the right laboratory tests are all that are required. Every doctor has picked up a case of anemia or low (hypo) thyroid state that clearly explains the patient's fatigue and lethargy. A vitamin B_{12} or folate deficiency can cause anemia, as well as numbness and tingling of the hands and feet resulting from a "peripheral neuropathy," or injury to the nerves of the arms and legs.

Unfortunately, there is no shortage of medical diagnoses, including cancer, that can present with fairly nonspecific symptoms such as pain, fatigue, and lack of appetite. But every situation is different. Obviously, if someone's symptoms have been going on for two to three years it is unlikely that cancer is the culprit. The cancer would have likely "declared itself" by making the person sicker and less able to do his or her normal day-to-day activities earlier on.

Once I'm satisfied that there are no hidden, lurking diseases, I can proceed. One is entitled to have more than one syndrome or disease. People with rheumatoid arthritis, for example, do experience symptoms of FMS on occasion. Depression can sometimes appear first, and then symptoms of FMS may develop. FMS does sometimes develop after a bad cold or viral infection. But if it's just that scenario, symptoms may slowly dissipate with time.

"Labeling" is a big issue. Some physicians worry that if they give a name like FMS to an undefined, blurry, watery group of symptoms, they are doing the patient a disservice. Such physicians probably don't feel that the diagnosis is credible, and they therefore feel that providing it actually leads to a worsened state of disability compared to how the patient was before the diagnosis was made.

No one ever questions whether giving the diagnosis of lung cancer to someone (when one of his lung x-rays shows a grape-sized tumor) is deleterious to the patient. Acne is just that. A broken bone is not questioned. We're not worried about "labeling" a person who had a heart attack, medically known as a myocardial infarction. But labeling someone with fibromyalgia is often questioned. This is pretty confusing territory for a patient and doesn't make much sense to me. It just reflects the continued unease with the diagnosis of fibromyalgia.

Receiving the diagnosis of FMS can actually be quite empowering for patients. Recognizing that they have a well-recognized set of signs and symptoms that is attached to a specific name can make them feel that they (1) have a "place" to go to, (2) can receive treatment for it, (3) have literature to read and (4) have other people with similar symptoms to talk to.

The diagnosis of FMS can make my patient feel less alone and rejected. A group of researchers found that providing the diagnosis of FMS did *not* cause a worsening of symptoms in the years thereafter. So "labeling," in my opinion, is not a bad thing. It can create a very good treatment atmosphere. Yes, some people with FMS may try to hide behind the diagnosis and not seek out the reasons for their illness. That's where a greater understanding of FMS's complexities and possible treatments can help. Too often, insurance bodies, workers' compensation boards, and other agencies "miss the drift," and therapeutic hell breaks loose. They may be reasoning, "FMS doesn't exist, or, if it does exist, it is a totally psychological problem, so why should we provide any disability benefits to the person who is experiencing it?" This may be faulty reasoning, but it's fairly common reasoning just the same.

Betty, with the foot pain and previous total body pain, got better because the physical and emotional stressors that were weighing her down lifted, and the tissues of her body were able to recover. The physical stressors included being on her feet all day, working six days a week, and performing all sorts of repetitive lifting, reaching, pushing, and pulling activities. Sore shoulders, an aching neck, strained calves, and LBG ("low back grumbling"—a term I just made up) are often the physical symptoms that result. Maybe exposure to warehouse-based chemicals had something to do with her symptoms, but this did not appear to be the case. The emotional stressors included the responsibilities of being a manager, overwork, and lack of time to spend with loved ones and/or in pursuit of athletic and leisure activities. In Chapter 1, I explain the effects of stress on animals' and humans' pain experiences and recovery from injury. Emotional stressors may in and of themselves become physical pain inducers by squeezing or contracting muscles, depriving them of normal blood flow and possibly pinching small nerves. Emotional stressors may also interact with any type of physical injury by impeding healing or causing central nervous system (brain and/or spinal cord) changes. Any painful stimulus may therefore stay longer than it should.

My "bottom line" is that fibromyalgia can be a result of several body system reactions to numerous physical and emotional stressors. Treat the body's responses—such as the sleep problems, the pain, the decline in strength and conditioning—and treat or attempt to resolve underlying social or emotional issues *at the same time,* and there is a fighting chance at recovery. Ignore the mind or the body factors, try to separate them from the treatment plan, and the chance of success is much lower.

Results as good as Betty's aren't always possible, of course. She may have had the benefit of being able to control her environment more than other people with FMS. Or maybe her fibromyalgia was still in its early stages. And maybe the rest of her life was rock solid, free of any significant financial, marital, child-related, or psychological issues. All of these factors can become very important treatment-related issues.

Let's now look at Helen's case and what she went through during her FMS journey. Her case illustrates more details concerning the syndrome itself, recovery, and the role of life events.

HELEN

Helen was 48 years old. She worked at a high-tech company as a middle manager. She had moved up the ranks over the previous 10 years and now managed about 12 people doing special projects. She described herself as a meticulous, action-oriented person who liked "getting things done." She was married for the second time and had two children from the first marriage. She hadn't been working for six months because of severe diffuse arm, leg, neck, back, wrist, and hand pain.

Where to start? Well, as I explained in Betty's case, not at first with FMS. Although the diagnosis was obviously on my mind, I had to focus on all the other possible diagnoses. I think that most North American doctors are pretty darn good at this point. They ask the right questions, examine the appropriate body parts, and order the correct types of blood tests and imaging studies. Sometimes, of course, too many studies are ordered, but that is the nature of our medical system. Every doctor worries about missing a diagnosis of cancer, and when a person is suffering so greatly from FMS, we tend to want to make really sure that there are no other treatable diagnoses.

Helen had already had numerous tests, including MRIs and electromyography needle probes. She was on vitamins E, B, C, and D, as well as chondroitin/glucosamine (chondroitin is produced predominantly from shark cartilage extract, and glucosamine is found in the covering of shellfish; vegetable sources are also available). Chondroitin/glucosamine therapy can be effective in some types of osteoarthritis, but in my experience it doesn't work for fibromyalgia. Helen was also taking large doses of acetaminophen and codeine (about twelve 30-mg codeine tablets per day). She had slowly worked her way up from two tablets "prn" (as needed). Her family doctor was obviously concerned about the amount of narcotics (the term used to describe the overall class of drugs that include codeine, morphine, and hydromorphone) but was perplexed about what to do. Physicians are repeatedly challenged to relieve suffering, and the subliminal or sometimes very overt message seems to be, "If the person is in pain, why not give narcotics?" I wish it were that simple. Usually, long-term narcotic use doesn't seem to be a proper solution for easing suffering, as we shall soon see, but, in the short term, when we're in the midst of managing so many other issues, narcotics have their place in the treatment armamentarium.

I asked about Helen's current level of activity. "What do you do on a given day? Are you active? Do you exercise?" Helen noted that she was a "slug personified," being much less active than she had been in the past. She used to walk her dog long distances in the bush, but now she took him out only to do his "duties." She used to clean her house like a whirlwind over a five- to six-hour stretch, but now she barely could get though an hour of dusting without having to stop, take a rest, and sometimes cry.

She had completely cut out any type of gym or fitness activities. Besides the inevitable experience of pain, she was frankly afraid of doing any maneuver—twist, turn, push, or pull—that might aggravate her pain. Even worse, she worried that she might be actually harming her bones, ligaments, muscles, tissues, whatever, by the performance of a specific exercise.

Tangents sometimes lead to the most interesting journeys and directions, and I can't not head off in a slightly tangential direction while we are looking at Helen's case and, in particular, her fear that exercising may worsen her condition.

The rehabilitation (e.g., physiotherapy, occupational therapy, massage therapy, chiropractic, kinesiology) and medical communities often talk about "hurt versus harm." This is a sometimes logical, often dangerous, way of think-ing that has the potential to both help and belittle the injured patient who is in pain. A physiotherapist's report may note, "I explained to the client the concept of hurt vs. harm." What does this mean? In its most simplistic sense, the phrase means "You can do this exercise—it may hurt you, but it will not harm you. So keep on doing it." Simple enough. We've all experienced some sort of back or neck pain and carried on with the activity we were doing. Some pain can be "normal."

But sometimes people can get carried away with the concept. A basketball player who sprains his ankle will have to do some ankle exercises that may be painful while they are being done but not after. Other exercises may cause severe pain that lingers over the next two days. I would say that harm is going on with the second exercise and likely not with the first. After certain neck and back injuries, a specific exercise may just be too painful to perform, and I don't want my patients getting caught up with deciding whether it's "hurt or harm." If it is very painful and the same pain lingers, it is likely that some harm may be occurring.

Patients with painful necks and backs may in effect be told they are not trying hard enough or that the exercise requested is not going to "harm" them. Sometimes that it the case, but sometimes it isn't. Every case must be evalu-ated individually. The injury, the person, the stage of the injury, the type of exercise being offered—it's complex, and just spouting "hurt versus harm" plati-tudes will not do the individual justice.

The yacht SS Tangent is now turning back.

Helen was becoming almost paralytic. She was very fearful of moving any part of her arms, legs, back, or neck. She worried that she was damaging important body functions. Keeping very still temporarily relieved her of some pain, but of course the pain relief did not last. Helen needed to move, and I'll discuss what she did and the role of exercise in FMS soon.

I asked Helen about her level of fatigue and whether she slept well. This is another huge area of FMS that deserves talking about. It is an area fraught with differences of opinion and, in my view, needless confusion. Excessive rumination about sleep and FMS is the result.

There are countless articles about the role of sleep in affecting, inducing, or aggravating FMS. Dr. Harvey Moldofsky, a psychiatrist in Toronto, Canada, led many studies into the area of FMS and pain. Disturbance in non-REM (rapid eye movement) sleep, resulting in the patient's waking up not feeling refreshed or restored (nonrestorative sleep), has been discussed, sometimes ad nauseam. Sleep is obviously an important issue to grapple with in FMS. But, as I've alluded to in Chapter 3, sometimes I feel that we physicians have "overcomplicated" the role of sleep. When you don't sleep well for a few days, you feel awful. When you don't sleep well for a few weeks, you feel like a mummy in a crypt. So, if you are worried about your child's health or the de-mise of your marriage or the fact you have bills that you see no possibility of paying, you don't sleep that well. And you start to ache. And if this situation is not somehow switched off, the disturbed body's sleep and pain systems start to falter and become larger and more menacing concerns. And fibromyalgia symptoms start appearing. Is that so complicated? The fact that more cases of FMS may have appeared as a consequence of the world economic meltdown of 2008–2009 does not mean that FMS is an economic problem. The huge stresses that resulted, however, may have led to numerous physical and painful symptoms in people from all walks of life.

The phenomenon of sleep deprivation and the production of pain was demonstrated in an experiment involving students deprived of sleep for two to three days. Once really sleep deprived, the students, who had experienced no pain before the experiment, started complaining of all sorts of aching, soreness, and annoying discomforts. Sleep disturbance is a miserable accompaniment of anxiety, depression, worry, unhappiness, or a death in the family. Diffuse or more focal pain in the neck or back is a frequent sequela of this sleep problem. There is some chicken-and-egg thinking here. That is, which came first, the sleep disturbance or the pain? The answer is that it is bidirectional: Either pain or sleeplessness can occur first, and understanding these associations makes it easier to understand what is going on in persisting pain or the pain associated with FMS.

Helen was in pain, not sleeping, and not moving much, and her employer was breathing down her back. She was receiving disability payments, but each month she had to submit a detailed letter from her doctor indicating why she could not work, and she felt belittled and devalued.

I asked Helen about sexuality, and the response was not what I expected. Usually when you're in pain, sex is not the first, second, or third thing on your mind. I generally note that it's not the pain resulting from a particular physical position that is the problem, but, rather, the lack of sexual desire as a result of feeling continuous pain and the often-ensuing unhappiness. My patients usually nod knowingly and seem to feel somewhat relieved by this discussion, and frustrated, too.

Helen wanted to have sexual relations, but her husband was reluctant. This was making her feel unwanted. It turned out that he was afraid that he would hurt her, and some counseling in this regard a little later on really helped the situation. In sexual health, the opinion of the complainant and the viewpoint of the partner participant are both very important.

The physical exam was better than I expected. There was no evidence of any red, hot, or swollen joints. Her neck and back moved slowly and deliberately, but they still moved. Arthritis or problems with joints did not seem to be the problem. She did not have the skin changes of psoriasis (a skin condition that is sometimes associated with a joint or arthritic condition). Her pulses were strong, meaning that her circulation was pumping blood in the right directions. Her reflexes, strength, and sensation—all components of the neurological exam—were excellent.

When I pressed the fibromyalgic tender points, 15 of the 18 were painful. She winced with each pressure application of my thumb but did not jump off the table.

546056

I thought that Helen met all of the criteria for FMS. She was diffusely sore, fatigued, and struggling and had the requisite number of tender points. Laboratory reports sent in by her family doctor did not note any problems with her blood, thyroid, kidneys, or vitamin B_{12} or folate levels. She didn't seem to have Lyme disease, a strange infection carried by ticks that, rarely, can present with symptoms similar to FMS.

It was time to begin our work together in earnest. I asked Helen to move her chair next to mine so that we could both see and work on the pain explanation and treatment diagram (Appendix).

I told Helen that we would first obtain an overview of her problems. We would then gather more focused information, and together we would decide which treatments would be best for her. There's no point in my just pronouncing my brilliant diagnosis. I was not going to be recommending a single surgical procedure or one shining magical pill as a panacea. FMS does not work that way, and, when you really think about it, neither do most illnesses. Medicine currently doesn't cure diabetes. It manages it, controls it, and provides education about it to patients and their loved ones. That's just how we try to manage and control FMS.

I did explain that FMS involves muscles and ligaments, not bones and joints. FMS was not arthritis, a bone fracture, or neuropathy. Sometimes even this information is helpful. I never say that the problem is in the patient's mind, because I don't think it is. A medical colleague reviewed one of my chapters and implied that pain is all "in the mind" and that I should change this fact throughout the text. Yes, pain is processed in the brain, and changes to the spinal cord and brain may make a particular patient more sensitive to pain. There are even instances where injury to a particular part of the brain, such as the thalamus after a stroke or the spinal cord after a motor vehicle accident, leads to the experience of a specific type of pain called neuropathic pain. But many other pain conditions are usually related to particular injuries or effects on specific body parts or systems. Migraine headache pain, for example, is a result of some disturbance (possibly spasms) to the vascular flow to the brain. Knee pain may be related to an injury to the collateral ligament (a tough band on either side of the knee), patella (kneecap), or other anatomical structure of the knee. Saying that all pain is in the brain may therefore be correct, but that just does not cut it for me. It just doesn't help me as a doctor or the person who is experiencing pain.

Helen and I started with general health issues and habits. An improper diet, obesity, cigarettes, and excessive alcohol use (see Chapter 6 for more about alcohol) can be a problem. Helen was not obese, nor did she smoke. However, she was starting to drink far more Crown Royal whiskies than she ever did in the past—two before dinner, one after. She knew that this was getting out of hand and indicated that she would be monitoring this situation. Social drinking with others, drinking wine with dinner as one means of relaxation—that is a practice that is perfectly fine. Drinking to change mood, using alcohol as a drug, however, is the wrong way to go.

Sleep was then discussed. Helen was waking up a few times a night, and when she woke up in the morning she just didn't feel refreshed. I pointed out to Helen, "You're not here in my office primarily because you have a sleep problem. Your pain, plus maybe worry and mood, has probably led to the sleep disturbance. But now the sleep issue has taken on a life of its own. If you are tired all of the time and feeling lousy as a result, it is hard to even approach the treatments we may want to try. We have to, in my opinion, 'treat the sleep.' That may be with hot milk or a hot bath or soft, soothing music, but it looks like you have tried those already. I think it's time to start a small dose of an effective 'sleep medication.'"

Most patients seem to understand my explanation and want to proceed. Others are dead set against any type of new medication. It bothers them that they may need to take a pharmaceutical agent. They want to be able to manage this sleep mission on their own. They are afraid of side effects. I nod and indicate that I understand but that "if we can string together a few weeks or months whereby you're more rested, feeling less crummy than in the past, then maybe the other treatments can be initiated. Maybe you'll actually be able to get out more and do the exercises that your physiotherapist has been telling you to do for the past 64 months."

I still prescribe amitriptyline, an old medication that used to be the number one choice of physicians for the treatment of depression. One brand name is Elavil, as in "Let's elevate your mood, let's put you on a pedestal. Let's. . . ." Don't get me started. Amitriptyline has fallen out of favor, and newer medications have taken its place to treat depression, ones with nicer names, marketed by attractive drug detail or pharmaceutical advisers, with apparently fewer side effects (maybe a few less), with profit margins that are much higher than the generic, pennies-a-pill amitriptyline.

I prescribe amitriptyline for its side effect of causing lethargy or sleepiness. Taken at around 8 P.M., at a much smaller dosage than used to be prescribed for its antidepressant effect, it's an effective sleep inducer and enhancer. "It's not perfect," I say "and that's the way I like it. It's a bit 'dirty' in that it has the side effects of dry eyes and dry mouth and sometimes causes trouble peeing, along with vivid dreams and, if you're unlucky, a too-healthy appetite. No one seems to get addicted to it because of these side effects, and when you don't need it any longer we'll just stop it. I'd prefer you take it nightly at first, but if you want to start if off just every once in awhile, that's okay, too."

Although amitriptyline has been found to help pain sufferers with neuropathy (nerve damage to, for example, the feet, often due to diabetes, alcohol, or unlucky genes) and other types of nerve-related or "neuropathic" pain (e.g., spinal cord injury, specific types of stroke, multiple sclerosis), I clearly state to my patients that "I'm not prescribing this medication for the pain; it's just for your sleep." At the small doses that I prescribe, it just doesn't help the pain of FMS, and therefore saying that up front makes me more believable. Too many MDs tell their patients with FMS that amitriptyline is a "pain pill." The patient gets disappointed when it doesn't work, and a lack of trust results.

Helen was game to try amitriptyline again. She had tried it in the past but was taking it later in the night and at much higher dosages than the 5 mg that I recommended. She therefore hadn't tolerated it. Of course, there are many other effective sleep-related medications that doctors may try, but I recommended amitriptyline first.

Next we talked about exercise and examined whether her level of exercise was not enough, too much, or just right. Not enough is usually the issue. Pain, a fear of moving, getting gradually out of shape, not working, feeling sad—all these contribute to not wanting to exercise on a regular basis. It's pretty easy to understand why this would be.

Helen needed coaching and some specific instructions about how she should proceed. I can't be an exercise physiologist, trainer, physiotherapist, and coach all at once. These people are experts in their fields and can help patients with FMS. But I can advise on how to get started.

Swimming is often a wonderful sport/exercise for people with FMS. Unfortunately, a substantial number of people are afraid of the water, don't want to see themselves (or others to see them) in a bathing suit, don't like swimming, especially the chlorine smell, don't have a pool nearby, and/or don't have the finances to pay for a pool membership. I keep learning about reasons why people don't want to swim, and I understand them all. It's also a bit of a pain to drag even an able body to a pool in the dead of winter.

Helen was game to try swimming. But that was not a guarantee that she would go. I have found over the years that it is necessary to give my patients a bit of a pep talk, some empathy, and understanding about this new swimming commitment. There is probably some psychological term for my "priming the subject" discussion:

You will have to start really slowly when you begin your swimming program. Baby steps. It will take you longer to drive or take the bus to the pool, undress, change into your bathing suit, and walk to the pool from the locker room than it will take to swim. Start only with one or two laps. Yup. That's it. That may even tax you too much or increase your pain. You may have to stick to one lap. Don't worry about it. You just want to slowly increase the number of laps that you do over the next three to six months so that you will eventually be swimming laps continuously for 20 to 30 minutes.

Over the years, I have noted that even these instructions are not enough. I have to instruct patients about which strokes to do. "You're not doing this to become a better swimmer, even though you probably will become one. You want to move as many muscles in your body and neck and back as possible, and swimming, with the water's lovely flotation properties, allows you to do that. Breast and side stroke, front and back crawl, moving the top leg and bottom leg in different sequences when you do the side stroke, back stroke, 'froggy style'—I want you to try all of these types of strokes. You'll do what you can and slowly progress."

The concept of swimming laps is sometimes hard for people to grasp. Aquafitness programs, available in many communities, often have a class specifically for people with FMS. They're great, they involve water's fantastic flotation properties, and I highly recommend them. Participants, however, don't swim laps, and therefore the ability of such programs to get people into better shape in terms of improving the conditioning of their hearts and lungs is limited. Swimming pulls, stretches, and sometimes tortures the FMS sufferer's muscles, but it's nice to know that at the same time some degree of aerobic fitness is being achieved, as well.

A recent study by Dr. Daniel Rooks and colleagues of Brigham and Women's Hospital and Harvard Medical School, in Boston, showed that "exercise eases fibromyalgia pain."[2] A structured exercise program that involved progressive walking and flexibility movements, with or without strength training, improved physical, emotional, and social function. Swimming, in my opinion, can partially achieve these goals, as well. I find that going to the gym can be a bit too much for some people when starting to exercise somewhat from scratch, but it's possible, too. It's the discussion, the initiation of the exercise, and then the goals—start slow and modestly, increasing weekly, biweekly, or even monthly—that are so important.

My physiotherapy, chiropractic, osteopathy, kinesiology, athletic training, and massage therapy colleagues may be critical players in the exercise focus of FMS treatment. Guiding and demonstrating the exercises, manipulating, treating, and massaging may all be major components of the treatment program. Asking me which is "better" is like asking which sports equipment manufacturer is the best. They all have their specialty areas. The key is that all of these disciplines should work together, sharing common goals and treatment plans. This rarely, if ever, happens and that is too bad. But it is just the way most medical systems currently work.

Helen said she'd try to exercise. I indicated that initially there would probably be increased aching and soreness but that as long as this "mini-flare" did not last long (e.g., more than a day or two), it would not mean that anything bad was happening.

So we had talked about habits, sleep, and exercise. Usually I then discuss the role of ergonomics, the machine-body interface, with my patient. This is more of an issue in the working individual, but people do a lot of work at their homes, as well—at their desk and computer, cleaning and maintaining their home and property, doing laundry, filling and emptying the dishwasher, mowing the lawn, shoveling snow, pulling weeds, tending a garden, taking out the garbage . . . the list of tasks that may benefit from an ergonomic assessment and help goes on and on.

I'm not an occupational therapist or an ergonomist; these are professionals who often deal with ergonomic issues. And these people should be consulted if at all possible. But it is not always possible because these individuals are not usually available in traditional health care systems unless you are an inpatient in a hospital. If you're an outpatient, they usually work in a "fee for service" setting, and many people simply can't afford them. If the patient has disability insurance or other funding for the services of an occupational therapist or ergonomist, I frequently write out on a prescription pad a request for such services, and that usually does the trick.

On a simple scale, I review issues such as pacing (e.g., cleaning the house or yard over a few days instead of a few hours). The computer screen should not be too low or too high. A decent chair can decrease neck or low back pain. Sometime even this type of simple advice can make a significant difference. Helen indicated that some of this advice made sense. She was already pacing herself to some degree, but whenever she felt the slightest degree better her activity level would zoom upward and pain levels would thereafter rapidly increase. An occupational therapist would certainly tell her that this type of behavior was deleterious to her health—that it was a "no-no," in simpler language.

Discussions about habits, sleep, exercise, and ergonomics usually resonate quite well with the "typical" (if there is such a thing) patient with FMS. He or she can usually relate to these issues and how they may aggravate, or sometimes even lead to the diagnosis and accompanying symptoms and signs of FMS. These issues are not too threatening, don't push too many personal buttons, and just make "medical sense."

Rather than plowing into the next category of functions or factors that can play a role in the expression or perpetuation of FMS, I preferred to ask Helen whether she knew of any other relevant issues. Usually if the patient has no idea what other factors may influence FMS, I'm in for a more difficult time. Helen offered "Stress?" as a possible factor, and I asked her what she meant by this comment. "Stress—you know, it tightens you up and can make the pain worse." I nodded in agreement. Helen was making some connections.

"Yes," I agreed. "Although I believe that FMS is primarily a physical problem involving muscles, ligaments, nerves, and probably the spinal cord and brain, psychological and social factors can worsen it and may, in some cases, be a major factor in the expression of FMS."

I then went on: "I don't know you, but as an expert in pain I have seen various factors play a major role. Here's just a brief list:

- Life in general
- Financial problems
- Physical abuse
- Sexual abuse
- Alcoholism—yours or a family member's, maybe a husband, brother, sister, mother, father."

These factors are printed on the pain explanation and treatment diagram (Appendix), and there are also blank spaces to fill in according to the situation. For Helen I added "driven nature, possible type A personality." I noted that any of these issues, and others, can play some kind of role in FMS. My job was to point out associations that sometimes, many times, people just don't make on their own.

Occasionally, patients react with anger to my list. They may say, "Oh, you think this is all in my head, that this is all stress and worry related." I have to head off this type of remark quickly, at the pass. "It's not for me to tell you whether psychological, social, familial, child-related, or other factors are involved with your pain. You have to tell me whether you think this is the case. I know that for many other people these are important issues to deal with even though the problem is a physical one. You tell me."

A few years later, I added a paragraph on the pain explanation and treatment diagram explaining why psychological and social factors were potentially important. Stress and anxiety lead to excessive muscle contraction and therefore can cause pain or a worsening of already present pain. Anxiety can lead adrenaline to flood the bloodstream, resulting in a rapid heart rate, excessive sweating, more muscle contraction, and more pain. "When you're already injured or in pain, difficult psychological or social situations can further screw up your pain and your ability to handle your pain."

Nowadays I may further discuss some of the mechanisms of pain discussed in Chapter 1 at the first visit or during another one. Chronic pain programs usually have an educational series of talks and lectures that discuss pain physiology, and they can be very helpful.

"Psychoneuroimmunology" is the science of the blending of psychology, neuroscience, and immunology. At its simplest level, one can distill it down to the following: When you're stressed, your immune system can be affected. You are then more susceptible to develop a viral infection or the "common cold." Wounds seem to heal slower. Recovery from illness in general may be impaired. I discuss many such possibilities, "mind-body" interactions, in Chapter 1 of this book and in an article published in the *Clinical Journal of Pain* in November/December 2008.[3]

The mind-body interactions in FMS represent a controversial and tough area but one that can't be ignored. Too often this issue is shunted to the side, probably because it's too threatening to both patient and doctor.

The questions that directly address the mind-body relationships in FMS include these:

- Is FMS an entirely "physical" disease without any psychological or social causative or contributing factors?
- Is FMS purely a psychological problem, a problem of perception of the patient and not a specific physical abnormality?
- Is FMS an entity in which combined physical and psychological factors and etiologies, attract, dovetail, and even cause changes to the other?

Obviously, my patients, and all patients with FMS, want specific, succinct answers to these seemingly clear questions. When Helen asked me whether I thought her problem was all in her mind, rather than summarize the entire world's scientific literature, I answered her as truthfully and insightfully as I could: "I think FMS is 'all physical.' I think that the pain you are experiencing is real, likely coming from some injury or change to your muscles and ligaments. You may have started off with a virus, overwork, or car accident, but, instead of going away, the painful symptoms have continued and increased. Some changes to your spinal cord, brain, or nerve flow, resulting from of feeling pain for too long, may be playing a role in the continuation of your FMS, as well. I believe that if we can together determine which factors are key driving ones, your FMS can get better."

I further went on to say, "I don't believe that FMS is a sentence to a life of pain. Psychological factors can sometimes be very important determinants of whether the FMS gets better. For example, if a difficult abusive marriage stays in the picture constantly and causes someone great grief, then this situation can cause muscles to twitch, go into spasm and fail to heal. If patients can do something positive for themselves, then I have definitely seen muscles get better and symptoms fade. It is not easy to change one's mood or life circumstances. But it can happen."

This is not always a discussion I like having because sometimes it leads to a type of confrontation that neither my patient nor I wants to have. There is often a lot at stake, such as commencement or continuation of disability payments, family relationships, and job termination.

Helen and I had talked for a long time, and it was time for her to go. Doctors' appointment times are rarely long enough for a new case of FMS. In the first place, it's usually not a new case—it's been brewing for months, and there always seems to be so much information to convey—that is, if the doctor is interested and asks the relevant questions. Which often just doesn't happen. Second, it's not always possible to zone in on one or two factors immediately. You may have to cover a lot of ground first to get to those key factors.

The whole process of explaining FMS and trying to make it relevant to the patient's life can be so complex and even frustrating. While many health practitioners may have been saying, "I don't know what you really have and don't really know what to do about it," the approach I have outlined is a bit more specific, and sometimes this is hard for the patient to handle. And, frankly, it can be exhausting for the caring health practitioner.

Helen looked a bit bewildered. She was, however, definitely going to try swimming, and she was going to seriously think about whether a psychologist could possibly help her. Work appeared to be out of the question for now. I would see her again in two months' time.

After Helen left, I thought about the issue of blame. Talking about social and psychological factors and their potential role in FMS or any painful condition can make patients feel as if I am blaming them for causing their own symptoms. This is a touchy situation. While I want my patients to feel that they have some kind of control over their situation, I certainly don't want them think that I believe that sheer will and perseverance will solve all of their problems and their FMS. After all, sometimes it was their driving, nose-to-the-grindstone personality that got them in trouble in the first place. I'd like my patients to leave the office feeling that there is hope on the horizon but that it may take changes to a number of work, home, marital, child-related, mood, and other factors to turn the FMS ship around. And that it is possible to do so. Slowly.

Helen returned for her 11-week follow-up appointment. Her pain was the same. She had started swimming in earnest, however, and was now up to 12 minutes of continuous swimming. She was very proud of herself and frankly amazed at her performance. At the beginning of her swimming program, she had experienced quite a bit of soreness, pain, and fatigue, but she soon got used to the experience and slowly worked through these symptoms. The main point was that, although her pain was the same, she was now far more active than she had been in about a year. This is an important point for all FMS sufferers: At the beginning of a recovery program, improving function and tolerance is more important than pain reduction.

Sleep was slightly better. She was taking 20 mg of amitriptyline per night. She had slowly increased the dose from 5 to 20 mg by 5-mg increments, every two weeks as directed.

Helen therefore felt a bit more rested, and with this new feeling of restfulness she was somewhat better able to tackle life's travails. She did experience the side effects of amitriptyline, the dry eyes and mouth and sometimes the increased hunger. However, she was prepared for these side effects and therefore did not feel threatened or disturbed by them. If you know your enemy, it can become your friend or at least an acquaintance that you can tolerate. Amitriptyline was being tolerated.

What about sex? Well, I had not discussed it much, but Helen realized that she would have to educate her husband about this activity. With her physical improvement due to swimming and greater pain tolerance, she convinced her husband to take a warm shower with her. Not a bad way to stimulate the juices of any couple. Her husband soon learned that he was not going to break his wife by engaging in sexual relations. Sex wasn't perfect, but Helen indicated that at least she was engaging in it. That made her feel more like a woman—more normal, and more desirable.

Helen was still thinking about the role or roles that psychological factors played in her illness. She noted that she had never really thought about how her hard-driving nature, her high level of anxiety, her sensitivity, and her need to "do things right" could be contributing to the diagnosis of FMS. She didn't really want to go there, as this mode of thinking seemed to negate the physicality of FMS. If psychological factors had something to do with her FMS, maybe it was all "in her head" after all. This was the message that Helen conveyed.

This is a tough dilemma. We talked about how complicated her thoughts and situation was. There were so many possible models. Her FMS had started around the time when her company was short-staffed and she was trying to do her managerial job as well as the job of one of her employees. She was coming home late every day. She was arguing more with her bosses and her husband. But she still wanted everything to be perfect.

Trying to be perfect under the best of circumstances is fatiguing. Trying to be perfect when the office was in disarray and understaffed and when there was a less than ideal product line created tremendous tension and strain. Time at the computer increased by hours a day. Is it so hard to understand that this situation gradually led to neck and shoulder pain? And poor sleep? And aggravation? And pain in the forearms, which slowly spread to other parts of the body, because she was now typing nonstop?

Where and when that critical line is crossed between being too busy, too harried, and too stressed and developing the signs and symptoms of FMS is not always clear. The answer "it depends" fits so well here. It depends on what is going on in your life at the time, whether your job, marriage, child's health, and personal affairs are going well. It depends on what went on in your life as a child: whether you had a warm, easy childhood, whether you were bullied or abused, whether you were listened to and respected. It may depend on so many factors. Some of these issues are discussed in other chapters in this book.

Helen had not yet seen a psychologist or psychotherapist. I thought that this could be a useful intervention, "to identify whether there are any barriers to rehabilitation." She agreed, but only after we discussed at length the effect of past and present psychological events on our bodies. Trying to find out *why* she was so hard on herself was probably a good start. I'm no psychologist, but sometime I feel like I'm practicing a new field called "psychoskeletal medicine" (instead of musculoskeletal medicine). Catchy. Maybe I'll use that in my next book.

By Helen's third visit, I had received two reports from the psychologist whom Helen was seeing once a week. Many issues were being explored. Helen wasn't very psychologically minded. Not many people are. The psychologist told me that she had to proceed very slowly. Issues with her mother were coming up frequently. And now her mom was dying from pancreatic cancer. There seemed to be unfinished business. Obviously, I could not become involved in these issues. I did say, however, that in my experience these types of problems could lead to many types of situations that eventually could lead to FMS. It was not a one-to-one correlation, but being stressed and anxious, perhaps suppressing many emotions, can lead to chronic muscle ache, soreness, and pain. Some people may develop chronic migraine headaches, others chronic back pain, and still others FMS. This is what I see in my practice. I can't always say why. Patterns develop and symptoms sprout up, and while one is dealing with the physical side of the problem, the mind must also be attended to. Mind-body medicine is probably relevant to at least half of all patients seen out there for many different conditions.

As Helen progressed with her new physical therapy treatments, she added massage therapy to the mix. This was a good sign. Initially, she hadn't wanted to be touched by anyone, and now someone was actually kneading her muscle dough.

Helen became involved in an FMS support group. Present in many cities across North America and Europe, these groups can be helpful and usually are. Helen felt that her particular group "grumbled and complained" too much. They grumbled about their pain and complained about their lousy medical care. In general, they were right, but she wanted to concentrate more on her wellness, so she stopped going. To each her own.

Narcotics stopped being a big an issue with time. Helen, with the aid of her family doctor, started to slowly wean herself off them once she started to feel overall better and more in control of her situation. She now took narcotics once or twice a week, rather than daily, only when her pain escalated to an intolerable level. I thought that was reasonable. Every person is different. She was also started on a new medication, pregabalin, which was approved in the United States by the Food and Drug Administration as a treatment for FMS. She thought the medication was helping.

After another six months Helen felt that she was ready to consider a return to work program. Yes, it can take that long. If FMS were purely a psychological problem, then possibly just the will to get better would fairly immediately dissipate its symptoms. But FMS is a physical problem and not purely a psychological one. Symptoms slowly improve as muscles and ligaments become less fatigued with minimal activity, possibly as hormonal, neurotransmitter, and body chemicals return to more normal levels. Sure, there is some speculation here, but this is what I see when I am treating patients.

But Helen could not return to the same job that she had left. Her psychologist, family doctor, and I all had to write letters on her behalf listing physical and psychological restrictions that were necessary to ease her return to the workplace. Every week or so she would do too much and crash. Her memory and concentration—the "fibro fog"—were not optimal but were certainly much better.

Helen was on a recovery path, but she wasn't perfect and probably would never attain the high energy and productivity levels she had before the FMS. But this time she did see a light at the end of the tunnel, and it wasn't a train coming her way. Sometimes the light shone brightly; other days it flickered and barely pierced the murky air. She hadn't "caught" her FMS as quickly as Betty, so a quick reversal of her symptoms was just not possible. Betty recognized the role that her life played in the production of her FMS symptoms and was able to quickly do something about it. Helen wasn't so lucky.

If FMS were entirely due to psychological, social, and coping issues, Helen would have recovered quickly or quicker. But FMS is not just in "the mind," and so even when the mind is better, the physical components of pain, fatigue, headaches, and lack of get-up-and-go can still prevail. These are probably the manifestation of the multiple hormonal, musculoskeletal, neurological, immune, and other systems that are affected by FMS.

Helen started to work part-time, and with a great new boss she managed to slowly build up her hours over three months to full-time status. Her new position did not require her to manage 10 employees. She could work more independently and didn't have to report to numerous bosses as she had before. Her struggle is certainly not over, but she understands herself better, and her family, boss, and workplace colleagues understand her situation better, as well.

FMS. Fibromyalgia syndrome. Tough. Hard to cope with. Hard to be a patient with. Hard to be a doctor for. But with a comprehensive approach, with treating individuals doing more than saying "get on with your life," miracles—or at least very positive life changes—instead of life sentences can occur. Dr. Jones's "glue the ducts" approach doesn't work for crying, and oversimplifying FMS won't work either.

If you have FMS, accept who you are, fight the fight, and get the help you need. You're worth it.

NOTES

1. "How Sad Songs Help Us Face the Music/Why Hurtin' Songs Make Us Feel Better," *Globe and Mail,* Toronto, August 2, 2008, p. R2.

2. D. S. Rooks, S. Gautam, M. Romeling, et al., "Group Exercise, Education, and Combination Self-Management in Women with Fibromyalgia: A Randomized Trial," *Archives of Internal Medicine* 167, no. 20 (2007): 2192–2200.

3. H. M. Finestone, A. Alfeeli, and W. A. Fisher, "Stress-Induced Physiologic Changes as a Basis for the Biopsychosocial Model of Chronic Musculoskeletal Pain: A New Theory?," *Clinical Journal of Pain* 24, no. 9 (2008): 767–775.

6

CHILDREN OF THE BOTTLE: ALCOHOL AND OTHER PAIN RISK FACTORS

There are many stories about my patients and their dances, romances, skirmishes, and down-and-out fights with alcohol. At the beginning of my medical practice, as taught, I would ask about alcohol intake whenever taking a history of any patient's illness. But I usually restricted the questioning to the individual patient's habits and behaviors. With time I began to recognize the immense role that alcohol played in some of my patients' lives as well as the lives of their brothers, sisters, fathers, grandfathers, mothers, grandmothers, aunts, uncles, and friends. And often it was not pretty.

This chapter first provides some background on the physical effects of alcohol. They are far reaching. I then discuss the concept of pain risk factors and demonstrate why a history of excessive alcohol use may be one of them. I have found that alcohol overuse by family members, notably parents, plays a substantive role in the presentation of my patients' pain problems. Alcohol is everywhere, and it creeps its way into many medical and life situations.

Alcohol has profound effects on virtually every system of the body. With high enough levels in the bloodstream, caused by prolonged and frequent drinking, the liver, kidneys, heart, and brain can all get hard hit. Pretty much everyone has heard something about cirrhosis of the liver; the liver gets hard and knobby and ceases to function properly. The liver is supposed to help absorb the fat in our food by producing an oily substance called bile. The liver is important in the breaking down of drugs that we ingest. Yellow skin, or jaundice, may result from liver failure, along with shifts in and out of lucid thought, poor energy, and frank flapping of the wrists and hands (I have heard it called the "waving goodbye sign"), or asterixis.

Nerve damage caused by the toxic effects of alcohol and brain injury causing dementia are other wicked side effects of "demon rum." Confabulation (talking fluently but making no sense at all) may occur in severe cases of alcoholism. The person speaks words without context. Sentences uttered are like a fragile necklace made of knots, empty spaces, and frayed string. And the beads are falling off in all directions.

With alcoholism, the pumping heart may become enlarged, beefy, and swollen (alcoholic cardiomyopathy is the medical term), thus leading to pump failure. The heart and lungs may become engorged, and congestive heart failure, or "water on the lung," may result. Cessation of alcohol use in such cases can actually dramatically reverse the toxic effects on the heart. The body can often take a lot of punishment before it goes down for the count.

How much alcohol is too much? In medicine, right from the beginning of our training we are taught a very specific rule about what patients tell you about the amount of alcohol they drink and what they actually do imbibe. *Double it!* If I ask my patient how many drinks he or she has on a daily basis and the answer is two, it likely means four per day, five means ten, ten means wow! that's a heap of alcohol.

It's not that we M.D.s are suspicious types—it's just that we have learned that it is difficult to trust alcoholic bearers of news. Does this alcohol rule-of-thumb always work? Of course not, but it does seem very accurate at times. And the goal is not to make a liar out of anyone but to get to the root of issues, concerns. and dilemmas that may intervene or be associated with alcohol and its many medical and social effects.

A glass of wine a day may actually have health-enhancing properties, as we read in newspapers and magazines. And it doesn't appear to be just red wine that is the magic ingredient: it may be an alcoholic beverage like beer, as well. Studies are not clear. Engaging in an activity that gives you pleasure and is not harmful makes sense as a means to overall well-being. How much is too much is still a question that remains. Alcohol to treat your mood or drinking to excess to escape it are obviously not recommended. Good judgment—not always available—is what is needed.

My patients in pain seek solace and physical relief. After they tell their story and the body parts are examined, it is time to assemble the puzzle pieces into the whole picture. Together, we try to establish links—across time, across places, with the past, with the present, with people, and with friends, lovers, or enemies. Alcohol-related issues are sometimes intertwined with these links, but not always. Alcohol may be a risk factor involved in various ways in the presentation of a painful condition. Let's diverge to the concept of risk factors and then explore alcohol's potentially diverse role in that regard.

RISK FACTORS

Risk factors constitute a major part of medicine. Risk factors are the events, times, factors, or forces that propel, or just barely ease you into a particular disease or illness.

Cardiovascular medicine (the heart) is a great example of diseases influenced by a patient's risk factors. Let's examine a heart attack (in doctor-speak, a myocardial infarction). A person is more likely to experience one if he or she smokes, has diabetes, has hypertension (high blood pressure), eats a lot of saturated or trans fats, or had a parent who experienced a heart attack at an early age. Therefore, smoking, high blood pressure, diabetes, and a family history of heart disease are all "risk factors" for the development of heart disease, such as a heart attack. This doesn't mean that everyone who smokes will be struck by a heart attack and die. But smokers face a higher risk that this event will occur.

So medicine and society spend quite a bit of time talking about *heart disease risk factors*. Television commercials and print ads try to convince you that if you take your blood pressure more often and ensure that if it is at the right level, by ingesting the proper medication, exercising, and watching your weight, you will be less likely to sustain a heart attack—very true! These ads try to find the right combination of sense, responsibility, and blood, guts, and gore to convince you that attending to your own risk factors will improve your quality and length of life.

Pain Risk Factors

One of my jobs as a physician is to help my patients find their own *pain risk factors*. Pain risk factors are not often talked about in the same way as heart disease risk factors, but they are actually very similar and definitely worth discussing. They are issues that are linked or associated with painful conditions. We should be teaching children and adults in society what they are. We may then be able to get a better handle on the prevention and treatment of pain-related conditions. Let's examine a few illustrative cases.

Sally had been experiencing neck pain on and off since she was 16 years old. She was now 40 and worked as an office manager. Pain came and went, but, over the six months before she came to see me, the pain had started coming more than it was going. As is often the case in so many people, stress aggravated the neck pain.

As I have said repeatedly, I can't jump to the conclusion that psychological and social factors are the main explanation for my patient's pain. Some combination of medical history, physical examination, laboratory testing, and imaging (e.g., x-ray, CAT scan, MRI [magnetic resonance imaging]) may be needed. It is only when comfortable with all of the medical information sought and provided that a physician can start working on a diagnostic and treatment model.

In Sally's case, the muscles and ligaments appeared to be the source of the pain, rather than the joints, nerves, and blood vessels that also exist in the neck area. Diagnostic terms such as muscle strain/sprain and musculoligamentous and myofascial pain are relevant ones here. The muscles were tender when I pressed on them. She had good movement, or "range of motion," but various neck movements hurt. These are all common findings when neck muscles and ligaments are injured and in pain.

The treatment plan then began. Together, Sally and I examined various factors that could exacerbate her pain. We started off with those listed in the pain explanation and treatment diagram (see the Appendix): poor sleep; improper ergonomics such as an ill-fitting chair or desktop arrangement; a lack of exercise; a history of smoking; and alcohol use.

Poor Sleep

Whereas poor sleep (discussed in greater detail in Chapter 5) may certainly be a *consequence* of a painful state, it may also be a *risk factor* for the perpetuation of a chronic painful condition. When we don't sleep, we feel fatigued, lethargic, and emotionally labile—our emotions are so close to the surface that they tend to spill out easily in response to casual remarks and the viewing of sappy movies. We seem less able than usual to cope with any emotional or physical threats.

Maybe some of the differing brain waves that accompany poor sleep patterns are also part of the reasons why poor sleep is a pain risk factor. "Treatment" of the disturbed sleep with a medication to prevent or reverse the development of chronic pain may therefore be necessary. Employing sleep-related suggestions that can be provided by social workers, psychologists, and family doctors can go a long way, as well. These suggestions, discussed in many pain manuals, include going to sleep at the same time every night, not lingering in one's bed, avoiding stimulants such as caffeine, and removing those negative thoughts, such as "I'm finished if I don't get a good sleep tonight." Not easy, but worthwhile.

Sally was not sleeping that well, and I prescribed a medication to assist in this regard. She also agreed to talk to her family doctor about "sleep hygiene," the term used to describe safe and effective sleep practices.

Improper Ergonomics

Poor office or general work ergonomics (the interaction between the body and its environment and tools it may utilize) is also a risk factor for the initiation or perpetuation of a muscular-based pain. Having papers far to the side of the computer screen (requiring the neck to be excessively stretched), having poor forearm support, and performing repetitive tasks such as 2,000 staple removals per day are just a few examples of poor work conditions. An occupational therapist or ergonomic specialist can help to establish a more efficient work environment.

Sally thought her office was well set up. She made sure, however, that any papers that she had to gaze at while typing sat right next to her computer monitor. There are specialized stands available that exactly fulfill this purpose. Buying one helped to decrease some of the tension in her neck muscles.

Lack of Exercise

Is being physically "out of shape" a risk factor for the development of chronic pain? I think so. Intuitively this makes sense. If you are not one to exercise, you may be somewhat weaker, have decreased balance, and have less breathing and heart power than a fit individual. Your potential for injury and for a rapid recovery from it are therefore lessened. Pain is a logical sequela.

Conversely, being in a chronically painful state often leads to inactivity, and as a result you become deconditioned or generally less fit. Your energy levels may be diminished, and a vicious cycle of less exercise leading to even less the next day begins. The risk factor of *a lack of or diminished exercise* rears its ugly head.

With Sally, exercise was virtually nonexistent. We talked about the need to do some type of regular exercise: swim or walk regularly, join a fitness club. "Yes, you can continue to bowl. If it doesn't hurt severely while bowling, and if your pain is not worse the day after, then it is okay," I encouraged. The emphasis was on the concept that "exercise may not change the pain, but if you are stronger and develop greater endurance, then you will be able to do more with the pain that you have."

Smoking

During the treatment-related session, I asked Sally, "Do you smoke?" I also often inquire about smoking when I'm asking about what medications the patient is on. After all, cigarettes are a type of drug. Smoking has been shown to be a factor in back pain. More smokers than nonsmokers experience back pain. No, it does not mean that if Sally stops smoking, her neck pain will suddenly disappear. If, however, smoking leads to poor circulation, because it causes atherosclerosis or "hardening of the arteries," then it makes sense that if muscles or ligaments are injured they will be slower to heal. Blood needs to enter into an injured area, clean up the debris, and create a favorable environment for healing tissue to be laid down. If the blood can't get to the injured area, it can't work its magic.

Plastic surgeons sometimes refuse to operate on heavy smokers, stating that they are concerned that wound healing will not occur and that complications are too predictable. If delayed or improper healing occurs, pain may not be far behind. So I consider smoking to be a pain risk factor. More and more communities are offering smoking cessation programs, and new medications to help people quit are constantly being developed. Quitting is very tough. Smoking is an addiction, and addictions are very hard to fight.

Sally had smoked 10 cigarettes a day for the past 18 years. "Worth looking into," I told her. She nodded. Now might not be the time to quit, but she'd been seriously considering the issue. She indicated that when she felt a bit stronger physically and emotionally, she would try to tackle smoking cessation. Her family physician had conveyed a willingness to help Sally with this task.

Excessive Alcohol Use

Sally's alcohol consumption needed to be quantified because, like smoking, excessive use is likely a pain risk factor. By affecting nerve function and by being associated with nutritional deficiencies (if you are drinking, you are likely to be eating poorly), ingesting too much alcohol may impair recovery from injury and lead to painful states. The association is not as clear as the link between, say, asbestos inhalation and certain forms of lung cancer. Excessive alcohol use, however, seems to be a risk factor for both pain development and perpetuation of pain following an injury.[1]

Sally was firm when she stated, "I don't touch the stuff, never have." *Sometimes,* my mind beckons to me, *such firmness means there is an alcohol issue lingering somewhere in the background. A family member, a parent, a husband. . . .* I didn't have to know right then and there. But I filed away this impression for possible later use.

Slowly, casually, Sally and I traveled through the pain risk factor towns of sleep, ergonomics, exercise, smoking, and ingestion of alcohol.

Psychological and Social Issues

It was time to look at a few psychological and social issues. I provided Sally with a list of items that "can, in my opinion, aggravate pain, or maybe even cause it to occur." These issues can therefore be considered pain risk factors as well. This was a venture into potentially uncomfortable territory, for me as well as for the patient. I always try to preface my remarks by indicating that "I didn't invent this list for you; I use it for everyone I see." Sometimes, but not usually, this allays some of my patients' anxiety.

My list used to stop after *financial worries, life in general,* and *physical or sexual abuse.* I was naïve. I didn't yet recognize that many life events could be responsible for many body chemistry interactions.

Financial issues cause anxiety. Anxiety leads to a potential cascade of central nervous system and peripheral tissue breakdowns, delays in healing, and other events (described in Chapter 1). This sounds pretty obvious, but it isn't always. To some insurance companies and worker compensation boards, a claimant's not having money seems to be a minor inconvenience. What I see is that not being able to feed the mortgage meter can delay recovery and lead to new mood problems such as depression, making the entire painful situation that much harder to recover from. Mental health, physical health—the whole mind-body script plays out as a consequence of lousy finances. A poor financial situation is a pain risk factor and is all too common.

Any negative life event—a divorce, a sick child, the death of a family member—therefore has the potential to contribute to physical illness and pain. Of course, we can take this statement and go overboard with it: *Dr. Finestone, you're just giving excuses for anyone to lay down and collapse into a state of vegetation. Who doesn't have issues?* Yes, there are many psychological and social issues out there, and not every last one needs immediate attention, but, then again, many do.

PARENTAL ALCOHOLISM IS A PAIN RISK FACTOR

Sam, another patient, told me about the support group for children of alcoholics that he was attending and how helpful it was to him. He recounted how cathartic it was to be able to discuss with other individuals what it meant to have a parent with a drinking problem. A penny this time barely squeezed through a slot in my brain. Not a total drop. Many other patients flashed before my brain.

I started to ask Sam about his childhood experiences with an alcoholic parent, as I subsequently asked Sally. Suddenly, explosions of information came hurtling at me. The information was difficult to hear.

The physical violence was one issue. Sally recounted how her father would come home blind drunk and break objects. He would then beat his wife, Sally's mom, and one or two of his children. He had favorites, like Sally, whom he rarely touched. But the violence was not what my patients seemed to remember the most.

Over and over again, I have heard how being the child of an alcoholic means being the victim of continuous uncertainty. Returning from school, Sam would never know which father would be greeting him at the door. Would it be the smiling papa, eager to help out with homework, discuss school events, provide a warm caress or a drive to the rink? Rarely, this father would appear at the doorstep. Would it be the sulking, quiet, brooding dad who didn't want to be bothered, who went upstairs to sleep, and who would come downstairs when everyone had already finished dinner and smoke and drink the rest of the night away without talking to anyone?

Would it be that totally inconsistent dad, the one who on one day would reward Sam for a chore well done but on another day, when the task was performed *in exactly the same way,* beat him for doing exactly the same thing, so that Sam would have no idea what the difference was? Would it be the dad who, coming home late from the bar, would rouse Sally and her siblings from a deep sleep and force them to clean out the garage, a chore that apparently he had asked them to do the day before? And if it was the mother who drank, would she be the one who never stood up for the children as they were being beaten by the boyfriend?

The uncertainty of the child of an alcoholic parent often produces terrible fears and, worst of all, a total lack of self-esteem. I have vicariously experienced the continuously rising bar that an alcoholic parent demonstrates to the child: one day, helping out in the home is enough, but the next day, it is worthless; one day, receiving an 80 on a math test is worthy of praise, yet on another day it is spat upon and a 90 is the only mark that will satisfy. The child is left standing in quicksand, continuously sinking in a pit of insults, profanities, and shame—growing up feeling worthless, of no value, contributing nothing to the health and well-being of the family. These negative values are perpetuated by some alcoholic parents, creating the risk factor *child of an alcoholic.*

My patients have expressed their ambivalence. They want to be the caring child, but they feel so used when they offer their help. When their estranged parent becomes medically ill, which seems to happen often, they rush to provide help with mixed emotions swirling in their heads.

Exposure to an alcoholic parent throughout childhood and, often, adulthood is in my experience a definite risk factor for the experience of pain and response to injury in adults. Lacking self-esteem and a warm feeling about oneself may lead to chronic unhappiness, anxiety, or a slew of emotions that I am sure the psychologists and psychiatrists have many names for.

Chronic anxiety leads to excessive muscle contraction, increased heart rate, fatigue, and many other symptoms. What I see is that, when the child of an alcoholic is subjected to a trauma such as a car accident, a fall down the stairs, or a sports injury, it may take longer for the injured part to heal. It may be harder for the person to cope with the injury and to bounce back. *"I am not worthy of recovering"* may be a message projected by the immune system across the cells of the body. This is just speculation, but I regularly see features of it in my practice. It also likely takes the presence of the other noted pain risk factors and many personal and social factors to produce a persistent pain state.

As I repeat regularly, risk factors are just that: risk factors. Having risk factors for a particular disease doesn't necessarily mean that you will get that disease. There are many well-adjusted people with alcoholic parents who are doing well in society. But, for the others, knowing this little bit about themselves can help them cope with or even escape from an escalating cycle of pain. Recognizing that being the child of an alcoholic is a pain "trigger" can help them start to remove the psychic weaponry that this risk factor can fire. They can, for instance, consider how their self-esteem affects their relationships with others. If I can connect with the patient and discuss this issue nonjudgmentally, then the next step—seeking help to start the process of emotional and physical healing—can begin.

Attending a self-help group for children of alcoholics, seeing a psychologist, social worker, or psychiatrist specializing in childhood trauma, participating in a multidisciplinary chronic pain outpatient program—these are the types of interventions that have helped my patients cope with being a *child of the bottle, a child of an alcoholic.*

Sally was stunned by our discussion. "So many thoughts are rushing through my mind, so many feelings. . . ." Alcoholism's effects are too often simply swept under the floorboards—even lower than the rug—and people have to fend for themselves in an area they do not understand. Help is available, but, first, recognition of the many issues involved is required.

Physical pain may accompany the emotional pain of being the child of an alcoholic. If the issues can be dealt with and some closure achieved, if a supportive spouse or family member can be available for comfort and caring, and if there are financial resources to pay for gym memberships, massage, or child care, as necessary, then positive results can indeed be achieved. Painful muscles start to unwind as anxiety and feelings of shame decrease. Strategies to cope with pain (e.g., medication, even if it has long been ineffective) suddenly start to work. Exercise, previously limited by pain, is now merely limited by the fatigue of doing it . . . and the body heals.

I have often flat-out told my patients, as I told Sally, that "you have been abused." Sally, in typical fashion, looked somewhat unhinged, puzzled. "Well, no, he rarely ever hit me, and there was never any sexual touching." There was such pain and guilt that she could not conceive that she had a right to express how she truly felt about the care she had received as a child.

"No child should be exposed to such violence, callousness and anger. You were deprived of a loving, caring childhood, and that is a form of abuse" is what I said, and I truly believe that this is the case. Hearing me say this seems to allow patients to relax, let their guard down, but sometimes only for seconds. The pain runs too deep.

Sally responded, although not immediately, to some of our discussion. She had to write a few things down, speak to her siblings (some of whom did not want to discuss the issue of an alcoholic parent), and talk to her husband and kids. She did eventually go to a self-help group for children of alcoholics and then moved on for some individual counseling. As usual, other attached issues concerning her own parenting and marital situation surfaced, but with time many positive steps were taken. And her neck pain lessened, becoming much less of a daily issue.

This chapter's winding and careening journey is almost done. Risk factors for pain include impaired sleep, poor ergonomics, a lack of exercise, smoking, consumption of excessive amounts of alcohol, and being the child of an alcoholic. And let us not forget the many psychological and social issues yet undiscussed. This is what I have seen, time and time again.

Message to children of the bottle: You can change from being adrift in the ocean, waiting for someone to pick you up and save you, to being a warrior standing tall and proud, protecting your loved ones, smiting the demons that drift by. The journey never really ends, but you end up the captain of your own destiny ship, rather than a passenger on the lower deck of despair.

Note

1. P. Latthe, L. Mignini, R. Gray, R. Hills, and K. Khan, "Factors Predisposing Women to Chronic Pelvic Pain: Systematic Review," *British Medical Journal* 332, no. 7544 (2006): 749–755; P. L. Brennan, K. K. Schutte, and R. H. Moos, "Pain and Use of Alcohol to Manage Pain: Prevalence and 3-Year Outcomes among Older Problem and Non-problem Drinkers," *Addiction* 100, no. 6 (2005): 777–786.

7

SHAME PAIN: I CAN'T GET NO JOB SATISFACTION

Can a workplace make you sick? Cause you pain? Short questions, very long answers. We know the answers are generally "Yes" and "Yes," but there are so many qualifiers. This is not the first story about work and pain, and it won't be the last. We are not dealing with a mathematical equation whereby work = pain. It is far more complex than that. Allow me to explain.

A fall from a faulty scaffold will render the window washer quite sore if he falls from a first-floor height. From the fifth floor, she will break a few bones and maybe suffer a brain injury. Falling from the twentieth floor? Death. The consequences of one type of workplace injury, such as a fall, can vary greatly.

A construction worker carrying too many loads of heavy bricks, an office employee typing too many reports while a fellow worker is on stress leave, a health care aide catching a squirming, falling, demented patient so that he won't fall to the ground, a youth counselor being kicked and pulled by a violent client: These events, seen over years of my practice, are workplace injuries that led to painful states.

It seems pretty clear that the particular injuries described led to the painful arm, neck, or back. What is not as clear is why healing and recuperation times varied so greatly in these cases. But now that you are more sophisticated and know about *pain risk factors* (Chapter 6) and the many psychological and social factors that can affect the pain experience, you are probably not that surprised by the differences in recovery times.

Sick-building syndrome—a state of feeling unwell owing to ventilation problems, construction materials, and other, still unknown factors—may be a workplace issue. The message from all this information is that there is much for the doctor to sort out when dealing with the worker in pain. Maybe the work doesn't even have anything to do with the patient's complaint. Maybe it does.

Lloyd's work and pain did appear connected. Circumstances involving the heart and soul were implicated. How one feels at work, and not just what one does at work, is this chapter's theme. Lloyd's is another mind-body tale that still resonates with me; it has further added to my understanding of pain in the workplace.

The referral note from Lloyd's family physician read "Pain between the shoulder blades, neck pain, tired of it all. All tests normal. Please assess and treat." A fairly typical referral to Dr. Finestone. Some of Lloyd's test results were faxed along with the referral request. I like when that is done.

I sat down with Lloyd. I asked about his age, marital status, number of kids. Fifty-four years old. Married for 30 years. Two daughters, one married. "Just trying to get to know a little bit about who you are," I said. People sometimes are taken aback when I ask such "personal" information. Maybe it's because we still look at medicine as a totally laboratory data-driven science where we plug in some values and poof! the diagnostic answer appears. I sometimes wish that it did work that way, but it rarely does. There is no substitute for a careful dialogue between doctor and patient.

My initial, casual observations were that he was wiry and fairly short, had a craggy face, and seemed uncomfortable, squirming in his chair, looking around, eyes opening and closing continuously. He just didn't appear to be a happy man.

More questions about Lloyd and his pain. "Where does it hurt, and when did it start?" He described aching, occasionally burning pain between his shoulder blades, or *scapulae,* and in his neck that had started about five years earlier. He was tired of it, wanted to get rid of it, and couldn't understand why it was still there.

There was no pain down the arms, meaning the problem was unlikely to be related to nerve root compression caused by a disc herniation. Many nerves leave the neck region (cervical roots) and travel into the arms. These nerves can be pressed on or squeezed for various reasons, including a disc herniation. In Chapter 10, I describe a disc herniation as being like the jelly leaving a donut (the donut being the disc resting between the bony vertebrae). Arthritis or overgrowth of bone around the holes (foramina) where nerves leave the neck can also cause nerve root compression.

Lloyd felt otherwise well, with no symptoms of cancer or infection such as weight loss, night sweats, chills, or fever. He had no bowel or bladder problems such as incontinence. I shudder to hear about bowel or bladder symptoms in any case of neck or back pain, as it can mean a more serious back issue, such as a spinal tumor. He had the usual few drops in the underwear after peeing what he thought was completely. That's likely a prostate issue—pretty normal for his age.

You have to rule out the serious medical conditions, Dr. Finestone. Not every case is psychosocial. My brain often gets after me like a whip. *You don't want to miss something important,* it tells me. *You're the doctor.* Thanks, brain. Medical school and residency training really try to create obsessive-compulsive doctors. That is good for the patients, but not all of the time—often you want that free-thinking, exploring mind heading your patient's way. Especially in pain-related matters.

More questions about the pain and its circumstances. "Around the time of the beginning of your pain, what were you doing, what were you working at, what hobbies did you have?" "Nothing . . . nothing . . . nothing."

This was like an attempt to find out the diet of an overweight patient. *What do you eat, when do you eat, how much do you eat?* Nothing . . . never . . . nothing. Of course, I am being facetious, but people's awareness of their dietary intake can be somewhat lacking, shall we say. Attributing events to a particular pain is a good idea, although the attribution may not always be right. It is a start on the pain highway. Lloyd did feel that pain mostly occurred during his work time. When I asked him to break the pain occurrence down into workplace:home percentages, he said 80:20.

"For so much nothing, you seem to be fairly miserable. What type of work do you do?"

He worked for the city. "I'm in an accounting position." "Do you like your work?" "No. Well, yes . . . no . . . not exactly."

Job satisfaction is important in musculoskeletal medicine. It's obviously important in any type of medicine: family medicine, cardiology, psychiatry, gastroenterology. If you're not satisfied with what you're working at, you're unhappy. If you're unhappy, muscles contract, the heart beats faster, the mind races, bowels loosen up or contract, and the soul fades.

A study sponsored by Boeing on back pain showed that job satisfaction was a risk factor for back pain chronicity. That is, a worker's back pain, occurring while the worker was riveting sheets of metal onto a jet's fuselage, could last longer and feel more intense if at the same time the worker's life was stressful, difficult, or awful. The back's chemistry behaved differently if one was sad, perplexed, angry, or dissatisfied with the job.

Low back muscle tension has been shown to be increased in distressed women. This may be part of the physiological issues behind the Boeing study. But the study was not really that well done, and it is probably inappropriately misquoted ad nauseam in scientific books and journals. The concept of job satisfaction and its relationship to pain chronicity makes much sense, however, and is worth talking about, doctor to patient, friend to friend, colleague to colleague. The study should not be used to blame workers for their pain. It does present some useful information.

Lloyd continued. "No one listens to me anymore. They avoid me. I've given so much, and I get so little. I should have been manager by now, but, no, the young guys get promoted, and they push me to the side."

The bitterness was rising to the top. He was so unhappy about his lack of recognition, his crawling instead of climbing.

He occasionally ingested Tylenol for the pain. Massage by his wife helped temporarily. Physiotherapy had been tried on and off on three separate occasions. Yes, he experienced some pain relief, but it was temporary. Sometimes the car ride home reversed the positive effects; sometimes the relief lasted two to three days.

It was time to take out the psychosocial shovel and do some more digging.

"Do you ever try to talk to your superiors?"

"They wouldn't listen. I have the skills, the ability, and they just didn't appreciate what I had to offer."

Lloyd was adrift in a sea of animosity. He was bailing his "woe is me" boat every hour, and the pail was always full.

He was so fidgety. He talked to me but didn't really appear to want to offer me much information. I was throwing my line into the water, and I was getting weeds, old shoes, and just enough information to keep me fishing. But it was tiring work.

Many patients can be leery when they are asked questions by the doctor. "You're the doctor, don't you know that already?" is a common phrase I hear. "You're the doctor, don't you already have that information in your files?" "Didn't my family doctor already give you that information?"

Well, doctors certainly send each other bits and letters and reports of information but not tomes of documents. And sometimes I'll receive only a quickly handwritten note saying, "In pain, please assess." And often doctors need to hear for themselves just what patients feel is going on with their bodies. So patients, please try to practice patience. I know, however, that the problem is usually tilted in the other direction, that it is the doctors who need to practice the art of patience.

Where to proceed? To the physical examination. Although the majority of information is often obtained from the talking part of the exam (the history), the physical exam can often offer up many pearls of information, too.

No matter how tired or stressed I may be that day, I have to do a complete job, just like the teacher, engineer, lawyer, or anyone else who provides a personal service. Patients appreciate a thorough physical exam. So many patients have offered, after my physical examination, "Thanks for spending the time, Doc, that's the first time someone has actually touched my back in two years." The application of the fingertips, the "laying of hands," is critical in my opinion, particularly in this impersonal world of ours.

Our medical world of tests—MRIs (magnetic resonance imaging studies), x-rays, bone densitometry, anal manometry, blood tests, urine tests, artery and vein Doppler tests, and so on—can be so impersonal. Of course, tests can be essential to the diagnostic process, but they may often be ordered so that the patient will not have to be examined. Ultrasound waves substitute for the palm of a hand or even the flat disc of the stethoscope. In North America, we've sometimes moved away from examining, and patients have noticed this trend. And often they are unhappy about it.

Lloyd smoked 12 cigarettes per day. This habit can cause narrowing of blood vessels, or atherosclerosis, as well as emphysema, wheezing, lung cancer, and angina. But I didn't notice any acutely revealing heart or lung problems when I examined his chest. His neurological exam—strength, feeling (sensation), reflexes, and gait (how the patient walks)—was fine.

I saw no unusual rashes, discolorations, or tumors when I looked at his neck. He moved it pretty well in the forward, backward, and side-to-side directions but complained of pain at end of range, or extremes of motion. This isn't indicative of very much, but certainly a sore neck could act in this manner.

His shoulders moved smoothly. He could clap his hands above his head, meaning that the shoulder pulley system, or *rotator cuff,* was at least intact. I did a few "special tests" of the shoulder, ones that are unique for this joint. There were no problems, but the muscles between the shoulder blades (or *scapulae*), called the rhomboids and levator scapulae, did hurt with motion and when I firmly pressed them with my thumb.

So he walked well and talked well but experienced pain when his neck and scapular muscles were moved and probed. He actually winced in pain when my fingers grasped these muscles and agreed that the pain was similar to what he experienced frequently at work.

There was no evidence of joint arthritis, no swollen abdomen (seen in patients with cirrhosis of the liver and those with bowel cancer), no numbness or tingling running down his arms. My mind kept running through lists of diagnoses. He had pain in the neck and shoulder blade area. The differential diagnoses, doctor-speak for the diagnostic possibilities of a particular case, were many: cervical strain, mechanical neck pain, myofascial pain, muscular ligamentous pain, soft tissue pain, parascapular strain. Mechanical pain is a nonspecific term meaning pain of the neck joints. Myofascial pain involves the muscles and ligaments of the neck. Muscular ligamentous and soft tissue pain are basically synonymous; both mean pain of the muscles and ligaments. Parascapular strain is pain involving the muscles and ligaments next to ("para") the shoulder blades. So many diagnostic names out there, but they all make sense, especially considering how many people in the world experience neck pain at one time or another.

Degenerative changes of the neck were seen on the x-ray report, but they weren't severe, and abnormalities of the neck seen on the x-ray aren't necessarily the source of the patient's pain. They didn't seem to be in Lloyd's case. If they were, his neck wouldn't have hurt primarily at work. Also, local tenderness is more common in muscular-type problems. His painful symptoms were coming from his neck muscles and ligaments.

What to do next? I took out my trusty pain explanation and treatment diagram (see the Appendix) and reviewed it with Lloyd. No, transplanting new muscles for the painful ones was not possible. Identifying potential causes, exacerbating and worsening factors, and treatments and remedies—that was our goal.

Like many of my patients, Lloyd was not sleeping well, and I prescribed a medication, amitriptyline. I informed him that it can cause dry eyes and mouth, increased appetite, and a hard-to-wake-up-in-the-morning effect. But it's a drug that has been used safely for a long time; it used to be prescribed a lot for depression. I mainly use it for its side effect of causing sleepiness. The side effect of a "morning hangover" is also present, but with careful attention to how much is taken and when (best time is about an hour and a half before bedtime), amitriptyline can have a positive effect.

If the patient has been prescribed amitriptyline already and has experienced difficult side effects, there are always other choices. If the person appears to be depressed, then an antidepressant medication with some sleep-inducing rather than energy-boosting side effects may be chosen. The family doctor can help me choose the optimal medication because, unfortunately (or thank goodness), I can't know every new or old medication. Knowing one's limits is important—in medicine and in life in general.

For Lloyd, exercise needed to be bumped up. Swimming would be an excellent choice as it seems to activate and exercise those aching neck and parascapular (next to the shoulder blades) muscles. Demonstrations of particular weight-lifting-type exercises that focus on the problem areas could be of benefit, as well.

Next, office ergonomics. The city had already sent over an ergonomic specialist to make sure Lloyd's desk and chair were at the right height, that his computer screen was in front of him and not to the side, that the keyboard fit his hands well, that papers were held close to the computer so that he didn't have to crane his neck to either side. Individuals who work for large corporations or government or nongovernment organizations are usually luckier in this regard. It's the smaller companies that simply can't provide the finances for such an in-house service. But freelance ergonomic specialists, often occupational therapists or people with a university degree in kinesiology, may be available to provide a private consultation. Ask your doctor to write down a prescription for such a service, and your employer will likely pay for it. I've done that for my patients, and it usually works.

Lloyd knew this stuff and fidgeted even more. "Anything else?" I asked. "Any other features or factors that could be aggravating your neck and scapular pain?" "Nothing I can think of" was his quick answer.

Now we addressed the last category of items on the pain explanation and treatment sheet: psychological and social issues that can aggravate neck and scapular muscle injuries or cause excess tension within the muscles. Or affect one's ability to cope with the ongoing discomfort. Or cause central nervous system changes that affect one's ability to "normally" perceive the pain signal. Or impede the body's ability to physically repair injured tissues, leading to a cycle of pain recurrence. This may not be the most orthodox of views, but it's one that has served me well in my practice, makes sense, and has been scientifically discussed in peer-reviewed pain journals.

Lloyd listened. Life, not enough money, sexual or physical abuse, alcoholism . . . "Any of these apply to you?" "Not really," he responded.

I filled in the available open slots with "workplace issues, they can definitely aggravate neck pain as well. Work-related tension, feeling unappreciated, feeling passed by. Those types of issues can be pretty powerful, Lloyd, in my experience." But his mind seemed to be drifting off. Perhaps he would rather hear something else.

"But what can I do about those things?" he asked. Good question. I don't always have the answers, but he is not the first person I have assisted with such problems. "Well, first think about them. Write them down. Maybe you can seek out your employee assistance plan, and a social worker can help you sort out some of those workplace issues." Employee assistance plans can be very effective early interveners in people's psychological and work problems. The social worker can often guide the client to the next necessary step of treatment.

Hmm. Maybe he'd done this before; maybe he didn't see a connection. Maybe he was just tired. It's certainly not easy to hear someone tell you to get help, especially if you're not sure whether the connections being made are accurate. And, of course, so many other personality, mood, marital, and family issues may be involved. What about them?

Lloyd didn't hear my unspoken musings, but he did reflect on my earlier comments. "My neck and work are connected? Can you fix my neck first, and then I'll fix my work?" Common questions that make lots of sense *if* you are not looking at the big picture.

The pain explanation and treatment diagram provides a near-perfect way to respond to Lloyd's unconscious (or conscious?) desire to disconnect his physical symptoms from the social and psychological world around him. Hey, we all try to do that.

I said, "Without the exercises for your neck and shoulder blades, you won't get better, because your neck pain is a physical problem. But without attention to workplace issues and your feelings about them, I don't think you can get better, either."

An analogy seems appropriate. "Sometimes we can look at the situation like gasoline and matches. If I'm in my office and there is a pool of gasoline on the floor, I can still work there. The room will smell, it will be unpleasant, and the walls may get a bit greasy, but I can still ply my trade for many more years. Same thing with a match. If I lit a match and threw it on the safety floor tiles, away from anything else, nothing would happen. The match would burn out, and I'd be on my way. I could continue working, no problem. But if I threw the match on the pool of gasoline, what would happen? An explosion."

I soldiered on, in an enthusiastic way because I really believed what I was saying. "The gasoline could be your neck and shoulder blade injury, the sore, torn, or strained muscles. Aggravating, painful, but manageable. You can cope with them, crawl along with them in tow. But what if the match is stress or bad feelings or a bad work environment? The combination with the neck pain leads to an uncontained blaze, a forest fire of emotions, regret, hurt, and heightened pain—pain that is now not tolerable, not contained, Lloyd."

Maybe this is a good analogy. For some it resonates, and for others it drifts out to sea. Maybe I shouldn't even have been getting into these types of issues on the first visit, and that is certainly a flaw of our medical system. People wait so long to see me. Maybe—well, undoubtedly—I try to ram too many concepts into the patient's head too fast. We doctors are often forced to provide this intense type of care. We don't bill by the hour, and our services are—fortunately for us but unfortunately for you—in demand.

I am aware that the ideas provided to Lloyd take time to process, and we all know that it is certainly not easy to change one's habits, beliefs, or circumstances quickly. It takes time and contemplation.

I told Lloyd that I would like to see him again in two to three months. He said he would take some time to think about what we had discussed. I prescribed physiotherapy to provide him with an exercise program. He knew about a pool program near his home and said he would try to sign up. The employee assistance program? A firm "maybe" was offered by Lloyd. There seemed to be indications that he understood some of our discussion.

The three-month follow-up date came and went. Lloyd did not show up. It was now eight months later, and Lloyd was back in the physical medicine and rehabilitation outpatient clinic where I work.

"How is it going?" Well, Lloyd had been busy. He informed me that three months after our visit, he had been discharged from hospital. Sudden chest pain had engulfed him about a month before that, and in the emergency department he was informed that he was in the midst of a myocardial infarction, or heart attack. He was rushed to get an angiogram (a picture of the coronary arteries, the blood vessels that supply nourishment to the heart), and the results showed numerous blockages. That led to urgent heart surgery, "CABG" (think cabbage), more formally known as coronary artery bypass grafting.

After his surgery he experienced the complication of a chest infection. The area where they split his chest open, the sternum or breastbone, was oozing pus, and he had to stay in hospital longer than expected to receive antibiotics and wound care therapy.

To me it was obvious. Tension, anxiety, worry, and lack of self-esteem, combined with smoking, which causes atherosclerosis (a disease in which plaque builds up on the insides of the arteries), all led to narrowing of heart blood vessels and poor to absent blood flow to the heart muscle, and presto—a heart attack.

And the delayed wound healing and infection? There is scientific evidence on wound healing and psychological and social factors that I wrote about in a recent *Clinical Journal of Pain* article. One paper discusses how "bacterial clearance" is reduced in stressed rats. The idea is that if a stressed rat's wound is exposed to germs or bacteria, the stressed rat will have a harder time clearing out the bacteria than a nonstressed rat. Nothing is ever that simple, but it made a lot of sense to me and for Lloyd's case. His wound, after all, did not heal that well and became infected, and he needed prolonged and additional care to deal with it. This could be related to his chronic anxiety, unhappiness, and absence of upward job mobility. Sure, this is speculative, but fortunately there is now plenty of evidence to back up these types of statements.

But something about the way Lloyd described his situation bothered me.

"By the way, how's your neck pain?" I asked. "Oh, it's all gone now," Lloyd said. Something inside me prompted me to ask, "Why do you think that is?" "I guess the surgery improved the blood flow to my heart, which increased the blood to my neck and shoulder blades, healed everything up, and made my neck pain so much better."

An intense silent scream started deep within the hemispheres of my brain, a kind of intellectual seizure, I suppose. *What? You mean you don't think that having a myocardial infarction got you out of your office, out of your stressful, miserable situation, thereby stopping all that adrenaline from spurting out of your adrenal glands and thus allowing your muscles to stop tensing and relax a bit, therefore stopping pain in its tracks? You don't know that?"*

But I didn't say that; I continued to listen to Lloyd talk about his pension, which would likely kick in now, and how he probably would not have to return to his dark and boring workplace and to the drudgery of his work among his apparently more deserving colleagues.

We've all experienced resolution of this or that symptom when another, more important life event occurs. Lloyd's cardiac bypass surgery did not allow for greater blood flow to his neck muscles and therefore less pain. But he thought it did. He had been stuck in a wounded mode until a more drastic life situation overwhelmed the less important job dissatisfaction, whether he wanted it to or not. His "shame pain" would likely return when another life event that he could not control came his way.

So physiotherapy or exercise or swimming or stretching or massage therapy or yoga or yogurt may be absolutely necessary to treating and healing the pain. But, as you'll be hearing from me over and over again, sometimes you need something else.

Like a specific action that cuts through your unhappiness, like a buzz saw through an oak beam. Like a change of jobs or a reduction in work hours. Like a move to a less stressful and maybe less prestigious position. Talk is cheap. Lloyd needed to stop blaming, start recognizing, and start doing something about his situation.

He was a cut-up turkey waiting to retire, get a pension, and "finally start living." But the next time I saw him, four months later, I saw a turkey that was looking far from stuffed. He had a strut and a grin that was contagious. Something had "clicked." Maybe it was the cardiac rehabilitation program, with its multidisciplinary care involving regular exercise and classes on healthy living. Maybe it was the smoking cessation. Maybe it was the supportive psychologist whom he was seeing weekly and with whom he could connect and finally unload years of brain baggage from his previously locked compartments.

"I think I get it, Dr. Finestone. I'm not always sure what it is I get, but it is about me, how I think, how I talk to my wife and children, how I react to others' remarks. Maybe I'm less of a victim; I'm still figuring it out." He was working at his job part time, deciding what was the best work path for him. Office staff, he perceived, were warming up to him . . . after all these years. From "I can't get no job satisfaction," he was inching closer toward the satisfaction side.

From shame to pain, to no gain, to reframe—Lloyd walked miles along these roads. Workplace factors were important, somewhat different from a sudden lift of a too-heavy object, and his heart surgery was certainly a peculiar way to deal with them. Other issues were important, as well, as they always are. Habits such as smoking, the psychological and physiological effects of chronic stress, distress and unhappiness, impaired sleep, an inefficient exercise program—all these had affected the health of those poor neck and shoulder blade muscles. It was, after all, their pain that had brought Lloyd through my door.

Lloyd was trying out new thoughts, walking down new paths to recovery, discovering what were his gas and match equivalents. It's never too late to pursue such a life course. Unless you're dead. And if you are reading this, I assume you're not.

8

CLENCHED FISTS: POSTTRAUMATIC STRESS AND FEAR

The effects of a traumatic event can be vast. And what trauma are we talking about? The bone-crushing hip fractures that occur when another vehicle comes slamming into ours? The searing back pain and sudden loss of feeling below our belly button, noticed after the car's three rolls into the ditch? Or the psychic trauma of knowing that, while we are unscathed, our baby in the back seat has died? The effects of any trauma may be confusing, disabling, disturbing, and . . . uplifting.

Uplifting? Before Brian's story is told, I digress to Dan and his traumatic event. Dan had his usual beer or three after work at the garage where he worked as a mechanic. He was heading home, late as usual. His son, little Albert, was six months old, and his wife likely needed his assistance, but "Hey, I can't do everything," he said to himself.

Dan had no memory of wrapping his truck around a tree. Maybe there was an oil slick; maybe he fell asleep. His left femur (upper leg bone) broke in half, and the orthopedic surgeon had threaded a shiny metal rod down the middle of the bony shaft—intramedullary nailing, in surgical lingo. He did well, went home after a few weeks, and now, one year later, he was back at work full time.

Dan was referred to me because he limped and was experiencing pain deep in his left buttock. I noted that he had weakness in the left buttock, or gluteal, muscles. Such weakness is fairly common after a rod is surgically inserted down a broken femur shaft. It is possibly related to muscle fibers or nerves injured as a result of the procedure or the actual trauma to surrounding tissues.

I told him what was going on and recommended a few exercises to strengthen the weakened muscles. Dan was pleased. "In spite of your accident, you don't seem to be too down or upset about your injuries," I said. "Dr. Finestone, that accident on the lonely highway was a blessing." "How so?" "Before that accident I was heading down a bad path, drinking too much, going out with the boys, not spending enough time at home. After the accident, my mind got clearer. I saw what a good, caring wife I had, the smile of my child, and how lucky I was to be alive. My boss was so understanding after the accident, and he helps me out if I have trouble with the lifting. Drinking is on weekends only. I am now way better off, even with my limp and pain."

So trauma + pain + limp ≠ unhappiness and disability. Dan had been dealt a deck of cards that another man might have scattered all over the place. Dan decided to order and realign those cards. Some were worn and frayed, but they were all useful and could deliver a winning poker hand once in a while. This is a reminder to us all that adversity does not always deliver bad news. But such was not the case for Brian.

Brian was referred because of "diffuse disabling body pain. Thirty-eight years old, married, father of two boys. He was involved in a motor vehicle accident and has never really recovered. He's seen lots of doctors and therapists. Any suggestions?"

In between my waiting room and the examination room there is a long corridor. Sometimes I call it my "private gait laboratory." A gait lab is a facility where the way people walk, limp, or even crawl can be studied. Specialized markers are placed on different joints, digital imaging is obtained, and all kinds of measurements are retrieved. Sometimes new, gait-related information contributes to a new understanding of the person's abnormal walking pattern—but not usually. Good eyes and astute observation seem to do as well.

Brian walked down the hall using a metal walker, very slowly, one foot shuffling in front of the other, with both shoe soles making a scraping, dragging sound. His head was down, eyes aimed at the floor. When he was about half-way down, I noticed that strapped to his hands, wrists, and forearms were white plastic slabs called splints.

Brian eventually made it down the hall and achingly eased himself into the office chair. Wincing facial contortions accompanied every physical motion. His balance seemed off as he moved from the walker to the chair.

I muttered to myself, "This does not look good."

Brian seemed to be suffering so greatly. The world, most of the planets, and a subsection of the Milky Way were pressing down on his hunched, defeated-looking shoulders. He rubbed his back and his neck with his splint-covered hands. He fidgeted. And, every once in a while, a low moan would emanate from his mouth.

Various reports accompanied Brian: the findings of previous consultations with a neurologist, an electromyographer (a doctor who specializes in diagnosing nerve and muscle disorders), a rheumatologist (a doctor who specializes in arthritis and/or joint-related problems), two physiotherapists, and a massage therapist.

I asked Brian what his occupation was. He was a flower delivery van driver. He volunteered that he had studied at college for a few years and had obtained a diploma in recreational management but "I never used it. We moved here, my wife got pregnant, there were bills to pay, so I had to start working. . . ."

His past medical history was uneventful. He'd had surgery to fix a broken nose years ago. He had fallen off the swing at a young age. He didn't smoke and drank socially, "a few beers once in a while."

It was time to take a history, the main event of medicine. The Super Bowl of the doctor-patient interview. This is where the doctor tries to understand what happened, what the sequence of events was leading up to the new illness, the sudden loss of vision, the seizures, the intense itching, the hiccups, the loss of feeling and power, the fatigue, the brown forearm spot, the sad feelings, the terror, the bed-wetting, or the memory loss. Symptoms, symptoms, symptoms, stories, wheat, chaff, doctor's interruptions. Remove, filter, keep, move to front of line—this is what is done with the retrieved information. This is what a history is all about.

Brian had been in a car accident two years earlier. While he was traveling straight through a green light, another vehicle, coming from the other direction, suddenly turned left in front of Brian's vehicle, a very common motor vehicle accident scenario. The front of Brian's bumper sharply hit the right front door of the other vehicle.

Brian volunteered, "There was a child in that front seat, Dr. Finestone . . . I saw her eyes . . . I saw the fear building up in her. . . . "

Oh my . . . I had heard similar stories before and my mind started to wander. Brian's tale was flashing forward into the future. I envisioned a pale, lifeless, dead 11-year-old girl—killed by Brian's bumper piercing the door's skin and crushing a defenseless child. I had dealt with similar cases in the past. Inadvertent homicide. Was that why Brian looked so sad and distraught?

"Was anyone hurt in the accident"? "No, everyone was okay. . . . The child was a little scared, but I think they took her to the hospital and then sent her home. . . ." Fortunately, I had been wrong.

But Brian seemed to be in deep distress. He spoke softly and made minimal eye contact. He frequently sighed. He was so troubled.

I requested more details about the accident. Brian was taken to the Emergency Department after the motor vehicle accident and had a few x-rays. The emergency record discharge diagnosis read "STI," meaning *I don't know what the hell this is,* or *I don't want to know what the hell this is,* or *He banged himself up,* or *It's not the bones, nerves or brains, but it is the soft tissues.* STI means *soft tissue injury.* Soft tissues? Read on.

I have seen patients who have been frequenting therapy clinics and doctors for months or years for a particular musculoskeletal problem, that is, a problem related to their muscles, ligaments, or bones. I'll ask them, "What do you think your problem is?" Often they will utter, "Oh, I have a soft tissue problem" or "My doctor said I have a soft tissue injury."

During the first few years of my practice, I assumed that my patients knew what they were saying and didn't question them. But when a patient asked me, "Dr. Finestone, what is a 'soft tissue' anyway?" I realized that the term was not well understood.

When I have asked the same question of my patients, I've heard, "It's soft, uh . . . like a tissue . . . I don't really know, but my doctor says it's a problem"; "It's like a tissue, I guess, kind of like a Kleenex in my body that got torn up"; "It's my muscles, I guess. . . ."

The last answer is the closest to being correct. But even doctors may have different definitions about what *soft tissue* actually means.

To me, soft tissues are muscles, ligaments, tendons, skin, and everything in between. Doctors usually know that soft tissues are *not* bones, nerves, joints, the brain, or the spinal cord. Sometimes, however, nerves—cord-like structures that travel from the spinal cord and snake their ways down arms, legs, abdomens, and other structures, supplying life, function, feeling, and power to muscles, arteries, veins, ligaments, and everything in between—are considered soft tissues, as well.

Brian hurt all over and was limited in how much he could reach, push, pull, sit, stand, and walk. He had not been working since his accident. He could barely help out with any home-related chores such as cleaning, cooking, or vacuuming.

A number of physiotherapy reports described a conscientious man who never missed his appointments. He'd achieved only minimal improvement in the neck, back, and arm pain, however. Many "modalities"—hot and cold packs, electrical stimulation, interferential current, ultrasound, intramuscular stimulation, stretching, and manipulation—had been tried, but to no avail. Acupuncture, with and without electrical stimulation, also did not produce any substantial relief. Brian was beyond frustrated.

Briefly, we talked about his background. He'd grown up in a small town, part of a family of seven. There wasn't much to say. "Pretty ordinary stuff, Dr. Finestone. . . . I worked hard, and I love my wife and kids. . . . Now I don't know what to do. . . . Can you help me?" There was a poverty of words, body motion, and thought. Brian was just hanging onto his life.

Money was a huge issue. For two years he had received 80 percent of his salary as long-term disability benefits, but the insurance company now refused to provide any further funding. The flower delivery company was no longer holding a job for him. His wife was receiving disability benefits; she had been involved in another motor vehicle accident and had suffered from chronic low back and neck pain ever since. Dipping into some savings was keeping the family afloat, but there wasn't much left. He voice reflected desperation. As noted in Chapter 7, financial stressors can become physical stressors, and any preexisting musculoskeletal issue may become worsened or aggravated a few notches. Brian's physical and psychological problems then expanded and crowded out any semblance of normalcy in his personal and family life.

Next step was the physical examination. His chest and heart sounded fine. Blood pressure was normal. I proceeded to the examination of the musculoskeletal system, following the bank robber Willie Sutton's rule, "That's where the money is."

Brian's hands were quite peculiar. He was wearing splints, which doctors and therapists call *wrist-hand orthoses.* An orthosis is any device that corrects or changes or accommodates a particular bony part or joint. Shoe insoles are *foot orthoses,* often referred to as orthotics. A back brace is called a *lumbosacral orthosis,* and so on.

I asked Brian to remove his wrist-hand orthoses so that I could get a better look at what was going on. He carefully and gingerly removed the orthoses by biting the Velcro straps with his mouth and pulling on them. Eventually, he peeled the splints off his wrists and hands.

His fingers had assumed a flexed, clenched position. Getting closer, I smelled a fairly foul, yeasty-type aroma emanating from his palms. I asked him to straighten his fingers out, but he could not. When I tried to see whether I could straighten out his fingers by gently pushing on them, he let out a yell. However, I gently tried again. I needed to see if a contracture or fixed deformity was present. This would mean that tissues around the fingers had solidified, making them impossible to move even with the greatest effort. A few degrees of movement were achieved, but it was very painful for Brian, and he buzzed and shuddered like a trapped housefly. It was hard to tell exactly how much actual finger movement was possible.

The pungent smell was coming from a few small cracks in the creases of his palms. The cracks looked filled with reddish-whitish material—fungus, I supposed. *How long have you had these cracks in your palms, Brian?* "Oh, a long time."

I wracked my brains to remember a conversation held with a plastic surgeon many years previously. I had seen a similar type of patient. There didn't seem to be any specific nerve, muscle, bone, or tendon injury. The plastic surgeon had nodded his head and said, "Oh, it's clenched fist syndrome . . . the guy's wacko. They hold their hands clenched, and it can get nasty because then they develop stiffness and contractures, and if a few breaks in the skin develop, fungus can get into that nasty moist palm environment and really go to town."

Sure enough, medical and Google searches yielded a plastic surgery paper describing *clenched fist syndrome* and hand problems that developed subsequent to a psychological issue. It's very resistant to treatment. The person holds the hands either tightly clenched, really closed, or in a state of flexion. Eventually, even though there is no actual structural injury to the hand's tendons, skin, bone, or joints, the fingers become stuck in a certain position, or, in medical terminology, *contracted.* This is what appeared to be happening to Brian's hands.

The rest of the physical examination revealed many tender muscles in the arms, legs, neck, and back. All movements were slow, deliberate, and painful. Bending over to pick up an object from the ground was a major challenge.

More information was needed. Brian was hurting in so many ways. He certainly did not appear "wacko," to use the surgeon's term. He was not in my opinion trying to be ill. I did not feel he was malingering, that is, feigning illness for his own gains. What gains? Living in misery? Of course, there could be many issues buried deep that could be affecting his recovery and healing. Malingering is rarely an issue in the patients I see. There are just too many other reasons and explanations for people's behavior.

What was bothering Brian so much? I had to find out more. "What goes on in your mind, Brian? Do you think of the accident often? Do you have nightmares about it?" Having nightmares and bad dreams about a car accident is fairly normal, but usually they last a month or so. When they continue to occur on a regular basis years after the event, it's a very troublesome and disturbing situation. It can mean that there are issues yet unresolved.

Brian regularly dreamed about maimed children, crushed heads, and bleeding bodies. Crashing metal, broken bones, crying scenes were all part of his nightly sleep, if you could call it that. He slept poorly because he could never remove from his unconscious the sight of bloodied injured children . . . defenseless children . . . children who could not be saved or protected.

There were a few psychology notes in Brian's file of medical papers. They talked about possible alcoholism in his dad. The psychologist noted that Brian was very hard to get through to. He met criteria for *posttraumatic stress disorder* (PTSD), a common psychological problem. War victims, police officers involved in difficult murder or rape cases and people who have been abused commonly experience poor sleep, fear, panic attacks, and a decreased ability to function in day-to-day living. Such people have been involved in a trauma that leads to a condition similar to the one that Brian seemed to be experiencing. Today's soldiers, dealing with Asian and Middle Eastern strife, are reporting PTSD symptoms like never before. It is likely that soldiers have always experienced such symptoms, but they were just never recognized. Armies and governments are finally coming around to acknowledging PTSD's devastating effects. Much more help is available now, but there is never enough, and it is still a struggle for soldiers to receive all the help, particularly psychological, that they require.

I could not engage Brian. He was focused on his hands. He said he was much better than he had been in the past. Now he could at least wiggle them a bit. The occupational therapist who had constructed the splints was so nice to him. This was important to Brian because he perceived that other treating therapists were less sympathetic. Brian's insurance adjustor was now treating him as a malingerer, "without any physical evidence of an injury." Those were the words of an independent medical examiner, an orthopedic surgeon who spent about 20 minutes examining Brian and thereafter made the malingering declaration. Brian was now falling to pieces. And I thought that this occurrence was a damned shame.

What was really going on in Brian's case? How could I analyze his painful situation in a caring, humane, and fair manner?

Brian was a simple, God-fearing man. He was lost. He had been genuinely physically hurt during the motor vehicle accident. He had trouble expressing himself. Maybe there were—I think there were—events in his past that led to this catastrophic reaction of heightened pain, clenched fists, nightmares, poor sleep, and no hope. He also was, however, experiencing a bona fide PTSD reaction to his trauma. Why did he react as if he had been involved in the murder of a child when in fact the child in the other vehicle did not get injured? I did not know.

What I did know was that Brian needed help. Unfortunately, he was being observed and treated in a piecemeal fashion, one part of him at a time. His hands, neck, and back were being treated by different practitioners from different branches of medicine and with different therapies. His mind and the feelings emanating from it were not being attended to at all.

Brian's whole situation needed to be evaluated by someone who had the time to see him daily for a few weeks—to check out his routine and his family life, find out how he coped, what made him tick. Surely Brian did not want to be living in this manner: scared, shaking, not capable of providing for his family. During this time he would require the finances to live like a human being, unafraid of financial penalties and pressure. Otherwise, there would be no point to this type of therapeutic exercise. A trained rehabilitation counselor or occupational therapist would be able to provide such a service to Brian. This type of individual, however, needs to be paid. Brian certainly didn't have the funds, and at this point his insurance company was not providing him with any funding.

I tried to talk to Brian about some of the psychological issues, but I just could not get through. Brian's car had penetrated the skin of another vehicle, but I could not get into his psyche. This made total sense in view of his limited psychological insight (probably similar to more than half of the population; we just don't talk a lot about feelings among ourselves) and his current desperate needs. It was quite clear to me that, according to Maslow's hierarchy of needs, Brian had to have food on the table and a sense that his shelter was being taken care of before he could start considering psychological issues such as those related to his PTSD. Maslow devised a pyramid whereby the lowest level describes our physiological needs: sleep, food, water, breathing. You need to have these before you can progress to the next level, a feeling of safety. Love/belonging, self-esteem, and self-actualization are the next levels. Brian needed to be guided through these stages. He desperately needed a psychologist's assessment and subsequent care. Many psychologists are expert in dealing with PTSD issues. They are skilled in slowly but surely counseling their clients, and I have seen the positive results they have wrought. It is a long process but, in the right hands, so worth it. Patients of mine have been saved from the depths of despair by a caring, competent psychologist who, working alongside other treating therapists, created the right healing milieu.

My assessment was that somehow, somewhere, Brian had to feel trusted and supported instead of hunted and burdened. I tried to convey these thoughts to him, but I doubted that much got through. Brian felt abandoned, and in actuality he had been left adrift. And his boat was traveling farther and farther away from shore.

As Brian left the examination room, I did not feel rewarded or satisfied. Maybe I had defined and validated his status a bit more, but he left as broken as he came in. His fists were clenched, but they were not in battle position, ready to get into the ring and fight. They were the hands of a beaten man caught in a system—in a maelstrom of past and present memory, of money troubles, of suspicions and hopelessness. And where there is no hope, there is nothing.

In cases like Brian's, the legal system is often the only recourse for improvement. It has been my experience that a competent, well-funded lawyer in conjunction with a supportive doctor and group of therapists can fight the system and achieve fairness for the case. Tempers cool down, the case is reevaluated, the recommended personnel are funded, and physical and emotional improvements start happening.

With a recommended treatment plan in place, we could foresee a brighter future: Brian's hands start opening, the cool air dries the moist skin, the anti-fungal cream starts to work, the psychologist feels that she can actually have an open dialogue, the vocational counselor finds Brian a volunteer placement, he starts to take walks with his wife and shows steady gains. Wishful thinking, maybe, but how can I continue as a physician if I don't at least occasionally experience such thoughts? My patients and I aspire to receive the best treatments available. Society then decides whether the treatments are possible. And so it goes.

9

ABUSIVE PAIN AND VITAMIN HOPE

Abuse. The term seems to be everywhere but yet it often seems misunderstood. Sometimes it is improperly used, as when a football player says he was "abused" by the referee when too many penalties were called. Most of the time we know what the term is, but we just don't like to acknowledge its presence. What is its relationship to pain?

Plenty. Every month I learn more about the relationship between a history of physical, sexual, emotional, or other types of abuse and the experience of pain. It's taken me many years to appreciate how a history of abuse can play a role in a person's overall health. It's obviously not a one-to-one correlation, that is, abuse = bad health outcome, abuse = pain. And there's not always a relationship. Some doctors roll their eyes when discussing abuse and ask me, "What are you going to do about it anyway, even if you know?" This is a very defeatist attitude that is not helpful to the patient and not demonstrative of an awareness of mind-body issues. Unfortunately, this type of attitude is not atypical.

And what is abuse, anyway? Here is a definition offered by the University of Toronto Community Safety Office: "A pattern of behavior in which physical violence and/or emotional coercion is used to gain or maintain power or control in a relationship. A single incident of assault also constitutes abuse."[1] In an editorial I once read, the author spent two pages discussing the definitions of abuse and how various professionals declare that it is both under- and overreported in society.[2] When a child or adult is regularly treated by another person in a manner that doesn't respect the former's personal, social, physical, or psychological integrity—consciously or unconsciously, purposefully or even without awareness—that, in my opinion, is abuse.

I once wrote a scientific article on the relationship between a history of abuse and pain.[3] A group of psychiatrists, a social worker, and I collaborated on a project involving women who attended a counseling group for people with a history of childhood sexual abuse. We compared their pain experiences with those of two other groups of women: hospital nurses and patients receiving psychotherapy who did not have a history of childhood sexual abuse. The nurses experienced quite a bit of pain, such as back pain; this is well documented in the occupational medicine literature. Overall, however, the women with a history of sexual abuse had higher rates of chronic diffuse pain and more frequent diagnoses of fibromyalgia and underwent more surgical procedures than the nonabused women. This is food for thought as we venture further into this chapter.

Women whom I have encountered in my medical practice, of varying ages and with varying complaints, come to mind. Through their experiences, let's explore how past and current abuse can influence the experience of pain. I will try to convey to you my understanding of the relationship between a history of abuse and the occurrence of painful musculoskeletal conditions. And try always to remember: You, the reader, and I are not looking at this issue so that we can find something or someone to blame; rather, we are trying to explain. Let's begin with Daphne's story.

DAPHNE

Daphne was 68 years old. She was married and had three healthy children and six vibrant grandchildren. She had been taking thyroid pills ever since she was told she had a "low thyroid" condition 38 years ago. She also had high blood pressure, or hypertension, which was well controlled by the medications she took.

Daphne was referred to me because of "pain between my shoulder blades and some low back pain." The pain had been occurring on an off-and-on basis for 10 years but lately was more on than off. The pain seemed to start years back when Daphne had pulled up the sod and tilled the soil of a large garden bed. She didn't take many breaks and had worked through the weekend. She couldn't rest much after that because she had all of her usual house-related activities. The pain never totally dissipated after that.

It was a burning, aching, sore sensation. Moving the arms and sometimes just sitting or standing would aggravate the pain. Daphne described the pain as feeling like tiny little daggers stabbing the area between the scapulae, the medical term for the shoulder blades.

Daphne had no peculiar rashes, no pain radiating down her leg in an electrical fashion, no weight loss, no fever or chills, and no trouble urinating or defecating. These are "red flags," serious symptoms associated with neck, thoracic, or low back spinal pain that one cannot leave alone and just watch grow. They can mean that there is a tumor, an infection, nerve root compression caused by a disc or other structure, or another serious condition. Doctors are taught to "root out" the red flag problems early because they often need immediate medical or surgical attention. She didn't seem to have any thyroid-related conditions such as slowness, fatigue, coarse hair, pasty skin, carpal tunnel syndrome (all seen in underactive thyroid conditions), or excessive sweating, racing pulse, or weak, aching shoulders (seen in overactive thyroid conditions).

Housework was slightly affected. She found mopping hard to do. She also found that taking care of the grandchildren was difficult; it was hard to lift those grandkiddies up, hard to diaper or bathe them. She had a few chores that needed to be done on her 1.8-acre lot. Her frail husband couldn't cut the grass, and she had taken over this responsibility. The vibration of the riding lawnmower was getting harder to take because of the upper and lower back pain that resulted.

Vibration from driving a car or truck or using a jack hammer is well known to cause or be associated with spinal, back, and neck pain. Truck drivers sometimes have a really difficult time with low back pain, and installing a hydraulic seat, which dampens vibration, can sometimes help. Some specialized seat cushions may help, as well.

Daphne was looking for some assistance. I asked about her activity level, and she declared that she was not very active in terms of sports or recreation. She was willing, however, to discuss increasing her level of physical exercise.

I asked Daphne whether she had any other concerns, worries about anything, about family members, husband, children, grandchildren. None. She didn't feel that she was depressed, but she did feel a bit "testy" now that her pain was more constant. This is a pretty common scenario—with more constant pain, the person is edgier, has less patience, and is less tolerant of people and events. My patients have described their "shorter fuse" as a result of their experiencing persisting pain.

I proceeded to the physical examination. Fortunately, she had few signs of arthritis. There were only a few bumps on the end, or "distal," joints of her fingers. Doctors may call these "Heberden's nodes." These are quite characteristic of an osteoarthritic condition, often called "wear-and-tear arthritis," not the more severely deforming types of arthritis such as rheumatoid arthritis.

Her neck moved well, as did her low back; however, she noted some pain with these motions. She was not experiencing much low back pain today. That happens. Spinal pain fluctuates according to how you are sitting, standing, breathing, thinking, and with myriad other factors. It does not mean that the pain does not exist. She reported tenderness on the palpation part of the exam, over the triangle-shaped trapezius muscles around the neck. The muscles aligning themselves over the middle of the neck and low back—the paracervical and paralumbars—were quite tender, as well.

When I pressed the muscles that attach themselves to the inner border of the shoulder blades, Daphne stiffened and winced. The muscles that attach to the shoulder blades are the levator scapulae (higher up) and the minor and major rhomboids. They properly position the scapulae when the shoulders and arms are moving and are used all the time with arm movement. Without muscles and ligaments holding the scapula in place, it would just fall down in a heap. Unlike other, deeper, fuller joints such as the hip joint, the upper arm bone (or humerus) is loosely attached to the very mobile shoulder blade. This permits much shoulder motion and freedom, but the increased flexibility comes at the expense of stability.

I recalled a number of past patients with similar pain and tenderness of the muscles attached to the inner border of the shoulder blades—an appliance repairman who suddenly had to reach for a washing machine that was tipping over, a victim of a car accident who had gripped the steering wheel so tightly that it actually bent on impact. In my experience, these shoulder blade muscles also appear to take a lot of "heat," meaning conflict. I often consider them to be prime "stress muscles," muscles that seem to react to stressful or anxiety-provoking situations more than other muscles, such as the biceps (Popeye's favorite arm muscles). "Carrying the weight of the world on one's shoulders" is a well-known expression. Worrying, taking on new responsibilities and shame all seem to place some added stress on those shoulder blades or parascapular (next to scapula) muscles, sometimes more than other muscles. This was something to keep in the back of my mind while I was trying to help Daphne.

The neurological exam, which particularly examines the nerves, muscles, brain, and spinal cord, was fine. No problems there.

But Daphne was in pain. She was not making her symptoms up.

History, physical, laboratory exams—the mantra of medicine, the ways we doctors must follow when diagnosing almost every case. Yes, sometimes a dermatologist can walk into a room, see the rash, and instantly diagnose shingles or herpes zoster without even talking to the patient. But going through the process of inquiring and then physically examining the patient and ordering any particular tests is still the cornerstone of medicine. I know I have mentioned these issues before, but they are an integral part of a doctor's and, therefore, a patient's life.

Daphne had already been subjected to a few x-ray procedures. Neck, thoracic, and low back x-rays showed "scattered degenerative changes." These types of changes are seen in people with and without pain. "Degenerative disc disease" and "osteoarthritis of the spine" are other commonly used terms meant to say the same thing: "The joints of the spine aren't perfect, but, hey, whose are?" or "There are a few worn, slightly broken down spots in your spine, but many people have them, and they are probably fine."

Are x-ray changes of a person's neck merely like wrinkles on a face, implying some type of tissue breakdown but not a serious health condition? It's often hard to know. The problem is especially compounded when degenerative changes seen on x-ray may actually *be* the source of the person's pain. Degenerative arthritis, the term used to describe some breakdown of the spine's joints, can be a painful condition but, as in so many aspects of medicine, not always. Go figure. Daphne seemed to be suffering more from injuries or symptoms coming from her muscles and ligaments, the ones I touched during the palpation part of the musculoskeletal examination. That was where I was heading on this diagnostic highway.

I left the room, Daphne changed out of her gown, and I returned to go over her assessment, the way I saw it. We went over the pain explanation and treatment diagram (see Appendix). The scenario to be described should become familiar to you as you progress through this book. First we had to talk about the diagnoses. Anyone and everyone is entitled to receive a diagnosis in response to the question "What do I have?" This is a serious matter that sometimes gets lost in the morass of terms that a patient is subjected to. Indeed, it's not easy being a patient. You may be diagnosed as having a "dysfunction" or "misalignment" or "strain" or "sprain" or "spasm" or "nodule" or "instability" or any of a number of other terms that are hard to define.

One particularly damning term is the pseudodiagnosis "pain syndrome." One of my colleagues especially loves to use this term. It implies, "Yes, the patient has something, but it's not something you can really define, examine, reveal, or see on an x-ray. I'm not saying it's in her head—I'm not a psychotherapist—but you know I'm not saying it isn't either. The pain doesn't follow any anatomy book diagrams that I know of, but, hey, the patient needs a diagnosis, so pain syndrome will do."

A pain disorder or syndrome "diagnosis" usually implies that there is more than "just" a specific pain in a localized or more diffuse body location. It implies that there are psychological and social factors that are the main, if not only, reasons for the pain. "Pain syndrome" sometimes implies that there really isn't much of a physical problem at all. But it does depend on who is using the term.

This is where the madness sets in—that because there is no history of a bone breaking, a nerve torn asunder, or an abnormal x-ray, and because "only" pain and muscle tenderness exist, some practitioners will say that there is no physical problem and that the real issue is indeed solely an abnormality of the patient's mind. It's another example of trying to divide and conquer the mind-body dualism of life and pain. Time and again I have observed important relationships among physical, psychological, and social issues encountered within my patients cases. However, starting with a physically based diagnosis, which I believe exists more than 90 percent of the time, is important to understanding the complexities of many painful conditions. Moreover, most people seem to need to know the physical aspects of their disease or syndrome in order to proceed further with their healing. Hearing "It's stress, you're okay" does not resonate well with many of the people I've treated, and the phrase seems to demean the entire health equation. As does using the term "pain disorder or syndrome," I respectfully submit. If the term if going to be used, let's be honest about what we mean by it: Pain that persists may lead to difficult social and psychological circumstances that, in turn, can prey on the individual physically and emotionally. That's a healthier explanation of a "pain syndrome."

We have wandered a bit off our trail down to the Grand Canyon of pain, but now we're back on the more traveled path, and I'm trying to convey to Daphne her diagnosis, words she can at least think about, relate to, and integrate into her healing program.

No one has all the answers, so I conveyed to Daphne a list of diagnoses that her history, physical examination, and review of her x-ray reports suggested: "The problem related to your neck, shoulder blades, and low back seems to be coming from your muscles and ligaments. Another term you may hear is myofascial pain, which means essentially the same thing: myo = muscle, and fascial = the ligaments and other tissue that hold and attach muscle to itself and to its anchor, bone. The particular muscles, those next to ('para') the scapulae, are called the levator scapulae and the major and minor rhomboids. Because the shoulder blade area straddles the cervical (neck) and thoracic (chest) parts of the spine, we can use also the more nonspecific terms cervical, thoracic, and low back strain or sprain." Sure, this is a lot of information, maybe too much. But at least it is written down and Daphne can consult it later. Or show it to family members or her family doctor.

I added, "It's also important to tell you what I don't think you have." The pain management and treatment sheet has a few boxes that I can check off in front of the patient. "I don't think you have a nerve problem. You don't have any tingling, numbness, or weakness, which we often see when nerves are affected. I also don't think that arthritis is playing a major part in your pain, but some discomfort may be coming from the cervical spine changes evident on your x-rays. We can't know exactly how much, but in my opinion those x-rays don't explain most of your current discomfort."

Daphne nodded. I pointed out the discussed muscle groups on the large diagrams of the body's muscle groups that are mounted on the walls of my examination room. This is pretty powerful stuff. Most people don't appreciate just how many muscles there are in the body and how big some of them are. We doctors forget that not everyone takes biology in high school or goes to high school at all and that knowledge of human anatomy is not that common. Knowing a little bit, however, seems to help, and I recommend to my patients that they look at any other pictures of muscles that they may see on the Internet or in library books.

Daphne was keen to know what she could do to improve her situation. I recited my usual spiel that "the best treatment would be to do a muscle ligament transplant. Take out the bad muscles, go to Costco or Home Depot, pick up the right parts, plug them into your shoulder blades, and away we go. Unfortunately, we can't do that in your case. Doctors can perform heart, liver, and kidney transplants, but they cannot transplant muscles and ligaments." For a quick second, Daphne pondered the seriousness of my remarks and then chuckled. Sometimes I do have to explain myself to a greater extent, especially if I just mention the transplant part and leave the conversation hanging there. Usually, the remarks go over well.

Daphne and I went over the other aspects of the pain management and treatment diagram. These include all kinds of issues that can "aggravate, worsen or delay healing of your pain." None of the first category of habits (diet, weight, use of alcohol, smoking) seemed to be a major issue here. Daphne volunteered that she might be salting her food too much, and I confirmed that, because of her high blood pressure, she should certainly monitor how much salt and/or salted food products such as pickles, delicatessen meats, and prepared foods she was actually eating. It turns out that many prepared foods, from soups to TV dinners to microwaveable hors d'oeuvres, can be superhigh in salt. Fast foods are usually high in sodium chloride, the chemical name for salt, as well.

Next up was sleep. She had never really slept well. I asked her whether she had any recurring type of dreams. I'm not sure why, but I find it is a good question to ask people in order to get some clues about their psyche. She remarked that she had vivid, violent dreams about people coming into her room at night. The individuals would just stand there. Sometimes it would be the same person, but she couldn't recognize him. Sometimes she would sense some type of death, but she couldn't be more specific. Daphne couldn't link the dreams with events in her life, or at least she wasn't telling me about any possible connections with past events.

When I was a young and foolish doctor, I would immediately try to excavate for psychological and social issues if it killed me, and likely the patient, too. I neglected to consider how that practice, during a first encounter, made it unlikely that a truly trusting doctor-patient relationship could be established. Just as in any other relationship, it takes time to develop a sense of security and comfort with your doctor. Then the information highway becomes a little faster and a little more efficient—the thought and feeling buses arrive on time and at the right place.

Daphne told me that she would periodically wake up in the middle of the night a few times per week because of her dreams, her pain, and, sometimes, a feeling of "restlessness." She took sleep medication occasionally but wasn't really concerned about her sleep pattern, and we decided we wouldn't "treat" her sleep with any new medication for now.

My diagnostic suspicion antennae were not really up; they were more "on guard," waiting for any other new information that might come. Violent dreams didn't necessarily mean anything, I reasoned, but why should she be having them? Although I am not a psychotherapist, my experience was that sometimes similar types of dreams symbolized distress. Distress and pain do frequently travel hand in hand. What was Daphne's source of distress? She wasn't telling me, for now.

Next was a short stop on the exercise or activity station. Daphne was not wholly inactive, but she agreed that lately she had probably been less active than she used to be. She would try to start walking again. I also recommended that she seek out a local aquafitness program or start swimming if she could (my thoughts about aquafitness and swimming are noted in Chapter 5). Last, I told her that I thought she could benefit from physiotherapy and massage therapy. Stretching and strengthening exercises were somewhat foreign to her, but she was willing to try them. She wanted to get better.

Massage therapy can be effective in many musculoskeletal conditions. We doctors sometimes have difficulties pinning down the indications for massage therapy for our patients. Insurance companies want us to declare that the massage therapy we ordered is therapeutic, that it is necessary to the healing of the injured tissue. It is not easy to declare that absolutely; there is just not enough research out there. However, I regularly see its beneficial effects in my patients. No, it is rarely curative, and it is not a substitute for active therapy and/or exercise, but it is a great adjunct to the overall treatment approach. Many athletes swear by their massage therapist. At the Olympics, massage therapists are busy day and night, kneading away. They are clearly part of a musculoskeletal treatment team.

Ergonomics, the machine-body interaction, was a bit of an issue. The riding mower was causing more pain, chores around the home were harder than they used to be, and maybe some adaptations needed to be initiated. Using a better cushion for the riding mower, doing less intense housework, hiring a housecleaner, and lifting the grandchildren less all might be useful, if not curative, suggestions. I thought that Daphne could benefit from an assessment by an occupational therapist, a health professional specializing in how the individual interacts physically or psychologically with the work, home, or other environment. There were not many of them available in her community, but perhaps Daphne's family doctor knew of such a local professional. Frequently, it is hospitals that are occupational therapists' chief employer.

Next stop on the diagnostic and treatment train involved explaining psychological and social issues. As I've noted in other chapters, I try to be as straightforward as possible in my approach: "I don't know you, and you don't know me. The habits, sleep, exercise, and ergonomics issues are very important. If we can treat any problems in these areas, we have a good chance at allowing the injured, sore, achy muscles and ligaments to recover. By taking away any negative forces on your muscles, you will promote healing and pain relief, and recovery is a very possible result." I believe these statements.

I continued: "The same holds true for psychological and social factors. They can aggravate, exacerbate and, less frequently, by themselves cause musculoskeletal symptoms. Some of the psychological stuff that I'm talking about is written right here on this sheet. Obviously, it wasn't written just for you."

The list is fairly long, and it will keep expanding as long as I am alive and continue to sprout grey hairs on my head and patients keep coming to see me. Life in general, financial problems, depression, anxiety, a history of physical, sexual, or emotional abuse, and alcoholism (in the patient or family members) are just some of the issues I casually bring up. There are a few blank lines that the patient and I can add to: our own "favorites." The reactions to this recited list may be incredulity, disgust, anger, a blank stare, a look of despair, a "what the f___ are you talking about" comment, emotional breakdown, mild to cascading tears, facial flushing, or what my psychiatrist friend and colleague Dr. Paul calls "the lower-lip quiver sign." Dr. Paul once told me that he had noted the "lower-lip quiver sign" in the course of his psychiatry practice. It could occur when the topic of physical or sexual abuse was brought up for the first time during a patient encounter. Sometimes the mention also led to tears and great emotional outbursts, but other patients tried to restrain themselves, displaying only a bit of lower-lip vibration. This sign has not been scientifically proved via careful controlled experiments; it's an observation that merely conveys the intensity of emotions that can result from the fairly casual recitation of

the list of psychological and social factors. It's an indication of the almost volca-
nic nature of our emotions. It tells us how feelings, secrets, and heartbreak can
be just beneath the surface and can erupt in a spout of anger, a flow of tears
and crying, or just the mild tremor of a quivering lip.

I like the list because it is offered in a truly caring, nonjudgmental manner.
Patients don't feel as though I am "accusing" them of any psychological or
social offense or transgression, and, if they do, it's easier to explain that I am
doing no such thing. Often the person in pain is truly tired of hearing "It's your
stress" without any attempt to link that observation to their pain and perhaps
to the core issues behind the stress.

But, as indicated, reciting the list can also provoke extreme agitation and fear
in patients. Perhaps I am just another doctor who is telling them that it's all in
their head. "What does abuse have to do with my pain?" they may say, overtly
or merely with their facial expressions. Anger may result, as well—directed
toward me or maybe toward certain past perpetrators or dark past encounters;
I don't know. I'm in the hot seat, trying to present information that I hope could
be helpful toward the resolution of their problem. In the beginning, what the
patient and I really want to do is find the common ground between us, a place
where we can share information in peace and a state of safety.

On the pain explanation and treatment diagram is another section that
explains how issues like feelings or difficult life events can play a role in any
person's pain. It notes that if stress leads to continuous muscle contraction
or tension, pain can develop. When you're tense, your heart may race, you
sweat more, and the whole pain experience is enhanced. And if you're injured,
imagine how difficult it may be to heal. I recounted to Daphne the story of
the injured mice (see Chapter 1): how a small wound took longer to heal in
stressed mice (mice that had been restrained in a tube, a condition that apparently drives mice crazy) than in mice that were free to roam about and receive
food whenever they desired.

Daphne couldn't relate much to the list. She had never really thought about
possible relationships between the mind and body. She did, however, find the
list interesting and could see how emotions could play a role in a person's
health. "That's a start," I thought to myself.

I reiterated that my job was not to judge anyone or force a particular label
or diagnosis upon a patient. In my experience as a treating physiatrist, I have
noted various relationships between the factors on the list and the subsequent
development of a painful condition. I told Daphne that if we could consider them
and get the right type of focus and treatment, positive results could happen.

Last, I told Daphne that if she thought any particular emotional, psychological, or social issue was of concern or relevance to her, she should speak to her
family doctor or give me a call. She could also search her own community,
perhaps the library, to see whether there were any mental health offices, self-
help groups, or other programs available to her. I have learned that the patient
must be involved in the selection of a therapist or program, such as a focused
group program.

If a person crawls into the emergency department of a hospital, bleeding to death and barely responsive, not a lot of permission or consent is possible or necessary unless the patient is a Jehovah's Witness or other specific group member and has a card in his wallet or health information bracelet stating that no blood transfusions are to be given for any reason. The doctors' first job is to find the source of the bleeding and to treat it aggressively. Later on, the treatment team may find out the patient didn't want to be treated, but that didn't really matter when the life-saving measures were started. The patient got excellent treatment that saved his life without his really being aware of what transpired.

This type of situation can't happen with "treatment" of psychological and social factors. Patients have to want to receive help. That's the only way they are going to marshal the strength and courage to enter the door of a self-help group or therapist. If health professionals, and society as a whole, could take away some of the blame by approaching these issues in a matter-of-fact manner and thereby allow patients to feel comfortable about dealing with their mental health or other issues, people would be much better off. Unfortunately, society is very far removed from this scenario at this time.

Daphne had a plan, and she was pleased. I did not detect any major angst or problems. She went home clutching the single sheet of the pain explanation and treatment diagram. My scrawl was all over it, and I was happy that she'd be able to re-read some of the points made during our discussion—if she could read my writing!

She returned three months later. She had quite a serious-looking facial expression, not unlike how she had looked when I first saw her. She sat down and reported that she was doing a lot more around the house and was swimming three times per week. Not bad. "How is the pain doing"? "Much better, but I have to tell you something." Daphne proceeded to recount a fascinating but awful story.

"When I went home after your examination, I thought a lot about our discussion and the pain management diagram. I have always been a tense kind of person, but I never really figured out why that was or how that could happen. I knew my grandfather had done something bad to me when I was a child, but the thoughts never all came together."

Daphne related a story of child abuse, perpetrated by her grandfather. It was a Saturday afternoon, the grandparents were over, and eight-year-old Daphne was playing alone in the living room. A glass and porcelain table lamp fell to the ground and broke into many irreparable pieces. Grandpa happened to be nearby when the incident happened. He seemed very concerned and spoke to Daphne in hushed tones. Daphne's interpretation of Grandpa's remarks was, "Don't worry, Daphne, I won't tell anyone. I'll buy a new lamp, and it will be our secret. You'll just help me out whenever I need the help—okay, Daphne?"

Daphne said that she didn't know who or where to turn to. From that time on, Grandpa requested sexual favors, which she felt compelled to fulfill. Oral sex and later intercourse occurred almost weekly for about four years and then suddenly stopped when she was about 13. Daphne described being in a trance for parts of those four years.

Neither her parents nor her siblings ever found out. Mom and Dad were loving, caring people. Daphne did well in school and married at age 21. Sex with her husband was somewhat hurried and not very pleasurable, but it was "not bad." She was always tense, and she always worried a lot about the where-abouts of her children and whether they were safe. She didn't make much of these facts, but now she felt that there was likely a connection to her history of abuse—childhood sexual abuse, abuse of power, abuse of privilege, abuse of the special relationship that exists between child and grandparent.

Daphne always carried in her a feeling of shame, of inner dirtiness, and she was really not sure why she felt that way. She never told anyone about her grandfather's terrible activities. She lived with the events, and I suppose because everything else in her life was pretty good—she was well fed, lived in a comfortable home, wore decent clothes—the consequences of the abuse were not as great as they might have been for people of lesser means. "And I would always feel an inner tension in my body, a feeling that my neck and shoulders were tight, that I'd just like to pull them apart if I could." Sometimes the tension in her shoulder blades and neck area translated into a headache at the back of her head, but it was never really a "serious" pain.

Only in the past few years, after she had been using her arms particularly vigorously, was the feeling between her shoulder blades more than just a ten-sion feeling: it was now an aching, sore, irritatingly painful sensation. Sometimes she wanted to just pull her shoulder blades right off her body. Sometimes it felt like a match was being held next to the muscles. I checked: no matches in the area. No lighter. No candle.

Daphne was telling me that she now realized there was a relationship between the tension she was carrying in her body and the pain she was sens-ing. She had never thought in such terms before. "So what does this mean to you, and what did you do about it?" I asked.

"Well, first of all, just knowing how my mind and body fit into each other seemed to make a huge difference." Daphne was exhibiting what happens to some of my patients. If the rest of their life is fairly stable and in decent order, they can focus on the relationship between the abuse and the pain. Daphne stated that she noticed a fairly dramatic lessening of the muscle tension sen-sation in her whole body when she forgave herself. She consciously talked to herself about her innocence in the whole sexual abuse episode, whereas formerly she had blamed herself and even labeled herself as encouraging or soliciting Granddad's activities. She was able to jettison all of those negative emotions onto the garbage heap of lies and bad deeds. These seemingly sim-ple acts produced a fairly immediate effect of diminished muscle contraction and pain. The two don't always go together, but usually there is a least some relationship. So many other factors, including the degree to which tissues are actually injured, what other stress is present in the person's life, other medi-cal diagnoses or injuries, and mood certainly play minor to major roles in the intensity and perpetuation of the pain. Fortunately, Daphne did not have many of these negative risk factors. (The concept of pain risk factors is discussed in Chapter 6.)

With the feeling of reduced muscle tension, Daphne could concentrate more fully on her physical exercise and conditioning. She was swimming for longer and longer periods and had less fatigue after completing her laps. She was more focused. Maybe that's what recognition of the roles that outside stressors and life events play in our lives does: it leads to understanding, to seeking help for oneself, to figuring out personal issues in greater detail, to better recovery and greater ability to recover from physical injury or illness. Daphne had genuine discomfort that was emanating from her muscles and ligaments, not from her brain. Her brain was, however, receiving the pain signal, and the brain appeared to be modulating the activity of her muscles and ligaments and possibly how the painful signal was perceived.

Daphne was learning how to manage her discomfort, and the physiotherapy, massage therapy, and occupational therapy all helped reduce her pain. Her painful symptoms did not all go away; she still experienced some shoulder blade area pain, but she estimated that it had been reduced by 75 percent, and she could now manage it much better. She could also recognize the physical and psychological triggers—too much housework, too much time spent on the riding lawnmower, too much worry about her children—and adjust some of her life accordingly. Of course, this could not be done all the time, and she was learning to accept this difficult fact, as well.

Daphne had moved from a state of powerlessness to a state of power. The childhood sexual abuse had robbed her of some of her self-confidence and caused her body to react in a defensive manner, with muscles always aware of the danger posed by her predatory grandfather. She didn't completely buckle under the pressure, but pain in muscles, ones that were needed to perform arm-related tasks, resulted. Now she could understand and accept the mind-body issues in her life, and she was investigating many potentially important topics. With her new sense of control, she felt less threatened, more in charge of the next treatment phase, the next feeling of useless shame, the next challenge. She would seek out counseling help that she felt appropriate, from her community library, a mental health clinic, her family physician, a community social worker, a private psychologist, a psychiatrist, a pastoral worker, a local self-help group, Internet sites, and numerous other possible sources. They all have the potential to be healing sources.

Let's now look at Tyra's story.

TYRA

Tyra's story highlights other abuse-related issues. No person's story is exactly the same as another's. We come to the table with different personalities, life circumstances, jobs, and relationships. Tyra's story of pain, body and mind, and her struggles to recover deserves to be heard.

Tyra was a 27-year-old single woman who worked at the airport as an air traffic controller. Immediately she related that she loved her job, the excitement of working in the airline industry. But she hadn't been working for more than three months, ever since she slipped on the tile floor of her bathroom while getting out of the shower. She was experiencing terrible back, buttock, and groin pain.

Tyra had never been ill a day in her life and had previously been very active, enjoying going out with her friends and engaging in rollerblading, and downhill skiing. When I asked her how she would describe herself, she answered that she was always "a fun, upbeat, happy-go-lucky" person. I find this to be an interesting question, and I'm still not sure how to interpret the many answers I hear. Most of the time people respond in a similar, very positive manner; people don't describe themselves as a "morose, sad, hopeless kind of person." Maybe when you're in pain, you don't even consider looking at yourself in any kind of negative manner. Maybe most people do see themselves in a very positive light, most of the time, even after an accident that has led to a persistent pain problem. Does persistent pain produce a bit of denial? Could be. People do want to present themselves in a favorable light, in general. Maybe that's a good thing. I'm musing, looking for these pages to jump up and provide me with some answers or clues. There's not even a twitch.

Tyra was beside herself. She wanted to be better, but she felt that her condition had actually worsened. Initially, her tailbone and buttock areas felt tight and fragile, "like a piece of glass." Over the next few days, she experienced more tightness, more grinding pain, more difficulty bending, sitting, lifting. At first she tried to just stay in bed, but this measure didn't help at all. This was consistent with a well-known study that showed that seven days of bed rest was no better than two days for acute low back pain.[4] Bed rest used to be a recommended standard treatment for back pain. Now it's just a given that bed rest for almost any musculoskeletal condition, back pain, neck pain, or ankle sprain is not a good idea. Recommending weeks of bed rest for a given musculoskeletal condition would probably be considered to be almost medical malpractice. But every case is different. Certain cases of back pain due to severe nerve root compression or fracture instability may need a few more days of bed rest than usual, but even this is debatable.

Tyra did not experience any back or buttock pain that moved, or "radiated," into her legs, the type of symptom one would see with nerve root compression. She didn't have any other "red flags"—no fever or chills, no bowel or bladder problems, no numbness or loss of sensation in her genital or anal area.

Tyra was attending physiotherapy treatments three times per week. The physiotherapy note said that she was receiving a whole range of primarily physical treatments: interferential current application, hot packs, transcutaneous nerve stimulation, some massage, laser treatment, and "mild adjustments." Her spine was maladjusted, not behaving itself. Tyra was trying to perform some of the recommended stretching exercises but noted, "I'm not getting very far with them. Going to the bathroom is painful, sitting is painful, and how can I ever consider bringing my knees to my chest, or trying to pull my chest off the ground while lying on my stomach?" She had a point, but still she needed to know that for back pain, movement is fundamental for recovery of the injured tissues, whichever they were. Tyra could visit eight different health practitioners—chiropractor, osteopath, family doctor, orthopedic surgeon, physiatrist, physiotherapist, alternative therapist, pedorthist (someone who makes foot orthoses)—and receive eight different diagnoses, interpretations of her signs and symptoms, and treatments. It's not easy being a patient. And Tyra was in a hurry to get better.

She didn't like to take pills. Her mother had, in the past, ingested too many Tylenol No. 3 tablets (which contain codeine), and Tyra did not want "to get hooked on them like her." She was quite forceful when she said this. A small red light, maybe yellow, went off in the right upper recess of my brain. Maybe I would get back to this later.

She recognized that her job was stressful but, as noted, loved it. I decided to defer any other psychological and/or social issues to the end of the interview. I needed to examine her and really try to figure out what was going on. When I handed her an examination gown, she indicated, "You're the first doctor to provide me with a gown; with the others I kept my clothes on." It's really not possible to adequately examine someone's back or pelvis while the person is wearing street clothes. But having the patient change into a gown does take more of the doctor's time.

Tyra was somewhat hard to examine because she was in so much pain. Just flexing (bending) her spine at the waist produced such severe discomfort that she had to sit down. But, as is often the case, sitting was even worse. Sitting generates greater pressure on spinal disks than standing upright. That's why you frequently see people with back pain standing around rather than sitting at meetings and shows. Tyra was actually bouncing up and down like a yoyo during the history part of the exam, sitting, standing, sitting, standing. . . .

Pressing the muscles of her back and buttocks sent "shock waves" of pain locally in the area. I could feel at one point a rippling sensation under my finger tips—possibly a spasm of the muscles, possibly a "trigger point," an area that some individuals feel occurs in many injured muscles. I'm not always sure whether I'm feeling a trigger point, but it seems like some people do have them. Some clinicians spend their whole lives treating trigger points, with injections of lidocaine and/or corticosteroids. The latter are not the same steroids as athletes take, and the amounts injected are small. Some doctors advocate dry needling (putting a needle in without injecting anything, akin to acupuncture), and others recommend compression with an external device such as a tennis ball. I'm no expert in the inexact science of muscle trigger points, but attacking the trigger points via multiple methods (e.g., exercises, stretching, compression with a tennis ball, and injection of lidocaine and/or corticosteroids) seems to make the most sense.

Tyra's neurological exam was normal.

Tevye the milkman was coming back to visit me. He's the "on the one hand, but on the other hand" guy in the Broadway play *Fiddler on the Roof.* On the one hand, Tyra's pain seemed muscular, but, on the other hand, she also seemed to be jumping out of her skin—somewhat out of proportion to her back pain, but how can one really tell? My gut was telling me that maybe, just maybe, psychosocial factors, past or present, were somehow at play here.

Plain x-rays had already been ordered and were normal. I did not think that an MRI or CT scan was necessary. I would have ordered these if pain were traveling down her leg or other red flags were present. Doctors don't need to order an MRI or CT scan for every case of back pain, but sometimes, because of this hyperlitigious society, we feel like we need to order them in spite of our past teachings to the contrary. In certain parts of sub-Saharan Africa, people with HIV infection don't have the cash to buy food, and yet they are supplied with retroviral medications. Meanwhile, expensive imaging tests of the back are being arranged, at times needlessly, in North America. As Bill Gates is said to have observed, who says life is fair?

Tyra and I sat down, and I pulled out the pain explanation and treatment diagram. She smoked, and we briefly discussed that. She was receiving physiotherapy, and I felt she should continue that activity. She was going to try to step into a pool to see whether being in the water could help her stretching capacity. Her sleep was disturbed, and I prescribed trazodone, a medication that used to be used for antidepressant reasons and is used more commonly today as a sleep aid. Tyra had tried amitriptyline and didn't appreciate the accompanying weight gain. At least she didn't have to deal with the truly dreaded side effect of trazodone, priapism, the medical term for painful erections. It rarely happens, but this side effect always lurks in the background when I'm prescribing this medication to men. Tyra was safe from this one.

Ergonomics was not really an issue at present. First of all, she was not working, and second, her chair and computer station were noted to be excellent; Tyra found them to be very comfortable.

I asked Tyra whether we could talk about her background, where she came from, her childhood. As is frequently the case, Tyra's eyebrows arched as if to ask, "Why do you need to hear about that stuff? I'm here for my back." I quickly volunteered that I was looking for information that could explain excessive muscle tension—stressors that would cause injured muscles to twitch more and cramp up and maybe even delay healing. She recognized that I was not simply being "nosy" or unnecessarily inquisitive. We both took a deep breath, and her story began.

Tyra explained that her childhood was not a smooth one. Her mother was young when she gave birth to Tyra, and her father did not stick around. She saw him once every year or two; they were not close. When Tyra was six, her mother remarried. Her stepfather was—to sum up in my words of interpretation—an alcoholic beast. He regularly physically and emotionally abused Tyra's mother. Tyra recalled that when she was 13, she tried to help her mom in the middle of one of her stepfather's drunken battering attacks. Tyra said that he—and I will never forget this—picked Tyra up by her throat and threw her against the wall. This was the first of many beatings to which she was subjected. In addition, he would constantly put her down, never complimenting her, never providing her with any warmth or encouragement. By age 16, she'd had enough and left home. Fortunately, she did well in school and was able to eventually land her current job as an air traffic controller.

The mother-daughter relationship had completely reversed over the years. Tyra now received distress calls from her mother at all hours of the day and night. The second husband was long gone, and Mom just couldn't cope. She needed constant nurturing and support. This was not easy to provide, as Tyra had her own career, relationships, and issues to take care of. It just didn't seem fair that she was saddled with the burden of her mother. But who says life is fair, Dr. Finestone?

Something clicked. Tyra seemed to "get" that all kinds of relationships could exist involving her mind, her social situation, her feelings, and her body. She educated me.

We discussed how being a mother to your mother was somewhat unnatural and agreed that this part of her life needed exploration. She had never thought about how holding in stress and anxiety could lead to all kinds of medical issues, such as headaches, abdominal pain, heightened muscle activity subsequent to a fall, delayed healing, pain escalation, trouble coping, sadness, and eventually depression, especially if finances became tight and disability insurance ceased to flow. Whew! This didn't all happen at once, but the tumbling-downward sequence of events made sense.

What to do next? I recommended some psychotherapy help. "Why a psychologist or social worker?" she asked. "What would they do?" Good questions.

In my experience, a competent, caring psychologist is worth his or her weight in platinum, for many reasons. They can provide a range of services:

- Providing a specific psychological diagnosis.
- Working with the patient to identify the core psychological issues that seem to be having the most impact on his or her pain and suffering.
- Educating the patient on the effects of a persistent painful condition on the patient and on his or her relationships with others.
- Role playing with the client (the term psychologists seem to use rather than "patient") to enable him or her to withstand the barrage of "What's wrong with you?," "You look fine—why aren't you working?" questions.
- Providing basic relaxation training and, if possible, more advanced techniques

This, of course, depends on the education and attitude of the patient. Some patients just aren't interested in the "psychological stuff"; it just does not have any meaning for them, and they can't relate to even the basic concepts. This may be a result of their culture, religion, or attitudes learned from their parents. It's too bad when it happens, because you just can't talk about psychological matters if the patient doesn't have any psychological insight.

A psychiatrist may be equally helpful, and there is the added advantage that psychiatrists can prescribe antidepressants if necessary. In most states of the United States and in all jurisdictions in Canada, psychologists cannot prescribe mood-related medications. Also, psychological services provided by a psychologist are rarely covered by government health services in Canada, while psychiatric services are. The same often holds true in the United States.

Some psychologists appear to really get stuck in cognitive behavioral therapy. All I can say is what my patients tell me: that cognitive behavioral therapy seems to deal with the here and now and with the symptoms attached. Strategies to deal with sleep disturbances and anxiety are provided in an expert manner. As for issues such as sexual or physical abuse, "I don't have the time to deal with those, Dr. Finestone; it's just not my thing" are words that have actually been said to me by a psychologist. These remarks may have been uttered because the funding insurance company would pay only for very goal-directed psychotherapy. There are all sorts of psychological treatments out there, and cognitive behavioral methods can be very effective. But it is my impression that in cases of past abuse, a more insight-oriented therapy approach is warranted. The overall message is that not all psychotherapy provided by a psychologist, psychiatrist, social worker, or other professional is the same. And that is another factor that makes it hard to be a patient.

Tyra accepted a referral to a psychiatrist, and we agreed to meet again in about two months.

When she returned to my outpatient clinic, her situation had improved. She was working out at the gym, very gently, and was planning to return to work. There was a sense of hope in the air, whereas previously there had mostly been despair. What had happened? "I went to the psychiatrist. He was nice, but I've only been twice. Mostly I went to my mother and told her I couldn't be her mother any longer. She was calling me three times a day, and I limited her to once every two days. I told her I loved her but there was only so much I could take, that stress and worry were making me sick. It was hard to do, but what a relief now that I've done it."

When I saw Tyra two months later, she told me she had successfully returned to work three days a week, Mondays, Wednesdays, and Fridays. She needed one day in between each workday to "recover." That makes a lot of sense and is the best way to return to work after a significant absence. Indeed, it's even better to start with half-days, then progress slowly to full days and so on.

Tyra soon recognized that she had had a lot bottled up inside her. She had channeled a lot of her past emotions arising from physical and emotional abuse into a healthy focus of education and career. Now was the time, however, to read books about abuse, get counseling, possibly join a self-help group, and really focus on healing and feeling better about herself. She continued to take many healthy steps along the way, with a few steps back on occasion, but she knew she could deal with her painful condition. By six months, the pain was about 80 percent improved, with only the occasional flare-up. She was much more open with her feelings, and her relationship with her mother was on a more even keel.

In my opinion, Tyra's history of physical and emotional abuse by her step-father and the poor quality of the mothering she had received likely contributed to her developing a chronic anxiety state. She could cope with these issues, but, with a superimposed painful injury caused by the slip on the set tile floor, her recovery was delayed and her injury was likely exacerbated. Her injured muscles and ligaments had a hard time healing. Her immune system may have been down. Her coping reserves then dwindled, and she didn't have the stamina or energy to carry on. Getting a handle on her abuse-related issues enabled her to restore her focus, initiate a personal rehabilitation program, and commence a healing journey. Her immune system may have started to function better, and the injured tissues began to knit together. Tyra's brain and spinal cord were receiving fewer emotionally negative messages, and in her calmer state, healing was more efficient.

Gertrude is the final person we discuss in this chapter.

Gertrude

Gertrude was a feisty 78-year-old owner of a local jewelry store. Quite a businesswoman, she also managed four properties owned by her brother-in-law. She was still plugged into her community, regularly attending board meetings of a local agency for the poor, even though her hearing was a bit reduced and her hip and knee arthritis gave her some discomfort.

Gertrude's issues were a bit different from those we've discussed earlier. She was experiencing low back pain, but it was associated with a feeling of instability, as if she couldn't stand without holding onto something such as a wall or the two banisters of a staircase. It was not vertigo, defined as feeling that the world is spinning, that the room is turning around you or that you are turning inside yourself. Vertigo accompanies inner ear problems. Scratch that off the diagnostic list. She wasn't fainting, she wasn't experiencing stopped beats of her heart, which could lead to sudden falling or "drop attacks," and no part of her body was violently shaking, as it would if she were having a seizure. Scratch heart and brain issues off the diagnostic list, too.

It was hard for Gertrude to explain, but we finally determined that she was experiencing a feeling of "freezing" or being suddenly unable to move, accompanied by a feeling of utter panic. She didn't know why she was experiencing such strange symptoms. Despite the fairly serious effects of these symptoms, she continued on with her life, trying to walk in areas with walls nearby, not walking long distances, driving to places as much as she could, and always holding onto the shopping cart when she was in a grocery store. She was a resourceful woman.

I had the benefit of reports from three other medical consultants: a neurologist, a rheumatologist, and an internist. She had had an MRI of her head and spine, multiple blood tests, and electromyography of her legs. Electromyography involves checking out how fast the nerves are traveling—nerve conduction tests—and putting needles into muscles to see how they are functioning and whether the nerves traveling to them are healthy.

All of Gertrude's test results were close to normal. Like many people her age, she had a few scattered changes on her MRI. She seemed sharp as a tack, and a diagnosis of stroke or dementia didn't seem to be relevant. Little "bright spots" in what is called the white matter of the brain are very common, and she had a few of these. Doctors used to think that they didn't mean much, that they were just part of the usual aging process, that they didn't portend any specific consequences. Now we know better. We know that people with high blood pressure, diabetes, or other disease may have more of these "bright spots" on their MRIs. Sometimes we call them "ministrokes." They may represent small areas of ischemia (or lack of circulation) in the brain. They may explain how one day Mom or Dad felt a little numbness or tingling in one hand or leg that thereafter dissipated. They may explain just a bit of progressive memory loss that happens almost imperceptibly slowly. And, in typical medical fashion, they may not explain much. My take was that they likely explained less than 20 percent of Gertrude's current balance or "freezing" problem.

The most striking finding on the physical examination was that if Gertrude walked toward me in the middle of the room she kind of waddled or walked as if she were on a tightrope. She held her arms out to the side and gently swayed back and forth. But she did not fall. When I had her walk down a hallway, her gait improved, and she attributed this stability to the fact that she could see to either side the walls of the long corridor. She preferred to use a cane just because it seemed to help with her balance.

Her back exam was benign. She actually bent and twisted quite well. Her muscles were not tender. Today was a "good day."

The neurological exam showed a slight defect in sensation of tuning fork vibration in her toes but not in her ankles. This was a possible sign that her peripheral nerves, the long strands of "wire" that travel from our spinal cord all the way to the tips of our toes, were malfunctioning. But she was 78 years old, entitled to a few frayed nerves in her legs. This finding couldn't, in my opinion, explain the severity of her described symptoms.

Once again I took out the trusty pain explanation and treatment diagram (see the Appendix). Not many bad habits to change. Exercise? She was reluctant or, rather, afraid to try much. Her sleep wasn't that bad, just somewhat fragmented, as with almost anyone over 39 years of age. You already know that a sleep disturbance can be an issue in exacerbating pain.

The list of psychosocial factors, however, produced a whopping number of potentially significant events. As a young child, she had been sexually abused by her brother for five years. She had told her mother, "but she did not believe me." It was her secret, and, except for one close friend, she had never told a soul. She had never gone for counseling, as "there was nothing available" when she was a child and she didn't see what counseling could do anyway.

Her husband had left her after 12 years of marriage for another man, and this had been quite devastating. Three of her children were married and had kids. The fourth child was a drug addict, unable to extricate herself from a swamp of cocaine, heroin, petty theft, lies, and deceit. Gertrude still talked to her but apparently had had to emotionally detach herself from this daughter to avoid the constant exposure to psychic pain. Gertrude cared about her daughter, but "too much, and it gets dangerous."

Where to begin? The obvious question to ask is, "What do these psychological and social events in Gertrude's life have to do with her feeling of imbalance and pain?" Or, "So, Gertrude has been sexually abused, left by her homosexual husband, cheated by her drug-addicted daughter. So? Many people have all kinds of terrible events happening to them, but they don't all experience pain or balance or panic reactions." I can't provide authoritative answers that explain it all. But in my experience, and as demonstrated in many articles in the scientific literature, psychologically traumatic events are "risk factors" for chronicity (persisting pain). The chapter on pain (Chapter 1) and my recent article in the *Clinical Journal of Pain* outline how mood states, particularly anxiety, can influence recovery from a wound and how stress in animals going to slaughter influences the quality of the meat produced.[5] Posttraumatic stress can cause headaches, stomach disturbances, pain, and myriad illnesses. Victims of disturbing battle related situations experience such symptoms, and terms like "Gulf War syndrome" have been coined. Past instances of abuse are traumatic events that can lead to future pain and health problems.

"I can't tell you what to feel or what is relevant to you," I said to Gertrude. "I know that in certain cases, with certain people, events like sexual, physical, or emotional abuse can cause or worsen many symptoms relating to pain. I have never really thought about balance, but when we analyze your complaints, they seem to involve freezing or panic more than anything else. It seems to me that being in a state of panic for hours on end would lead to many health problems. But you must talk to me about what issues may be key to you."

Gertrude seemed to understand but obviously was a bit perplexed. I wrote to her family doctor about my findings. I noted that, while she may have mild elements of peripheral neuropathy (diffuse injury to nerves at ends of legs and arms) and/or ministrokes, these two diagnoses did not seem to explain all of her symptoms. I asked Gertrude to try to increase her level of activity by joining a seniors' exercise program in her community. She liked that idea. I also asked her to think about any possible relationship between past childhood and adult events and her current situation.

Gertrude was scheduled to return for a three-month follow-up visit, but she missed her appointment and didn't reschedule. I didn't push the situation as, after all, I was trying to help her, not force her into a particular category or down a path she just didn't want to go down. People sometimes really need to think about the factors that may be affecting them. That can take a lot of time—months, years. Sometimes, it never happens.

About one year later, a new consultation request was faxed to my office on behalf of Gertrude by her family doctor. "Gertrude thought your administrations last year were helpful, and she wants to see you again." Why not?

Nothing had really changed. Gertrude continued to have difficulty walking in open areas and tried to restrict herself to stairways, hallways, her car, and shopping carts. She always brought a cane along to the community meetings she was involved in as a volunteer. She told me that she had been thinking a lot about our conversation and wanted to do something about dealing with her past. "What should I do, Dr. Finestone?"

We went over some of the difficult details of her past. "Anything else you want to tell me, Gertrude?" "Well, I keep remembering that I was thrown up in the air by my neighbors. I was the youngest child, and I remember how my mother would scream in fear to put me down, that I would be hurt by their lifting. I was so scared that I would be dropped in mid-air and break my bones, hurt myself badly." Gertrude recounted how this memory was with her constantly. It seemed that it was with her when she walked almost anywhere. It seemed like she was "freezing" in midstep, remembering her feeling of lack of control when she was tossed up in the air by her neighbors.

The mind can be tremendously powerful. Despite her successful life, her ability to provide for herself into her late seventies, her continued community action support, she was bending under the weight of past events, in my opinion. She was panicking to such a degree that she actually felt that she always needed to hold on to or see something close to her. But, for the first time in her life, she was recognizing relationships that linked the sexual abuse, her childhood, her marriage, her daughter's drug illness, and her life. She wasn't sure what they were, and I certainly wasn't sure, either. What we could do was try to provide her with some recovery tools so that she could find her way out of the deep psychological and physical pit that she appeared to be in. This time she was extremely game to try, and that made my job so much easier. "I am ready to take the necessary steps, Dr. Finestone. I may be old, but I'm not done yet."

While she also experienced some low back pain, it was fairly minor, more of a nagging nuisance type of discomfort. We decided that we'd attack both the pain and the "balance disorder" (nice medical term for "Help, I'm falling") with the same brush strokes. Gertrude required a mind-body approach. She had physical and psychological issues that needed to be addressed simultaneously. Yoga was a great tool for her to learn and practice. Stilling the mind, stretching, calming down—all seemed to be excellent goals, and yoga, I thought, could help her to achieve them. Yoga classes are now widely available in many communities, and people of all ages are participating. I don't think it's just a fad. It's not a complete treatment for any one problem. But what is? It's a useful practice that can help athletes of any type and stressed-out regular folk, and I can certainly understand why it's an everyday Hindu practice. What's wrong with focusing on relaxing the mind to eventually help solve personal or world-related issues? And improving flexibility, which yoga can help achieve, is likely beneficial to those who participate in any sporting, hobby, or household chore activity.

Next, a psychologist or social worker needed to be engaged to help Gertrude sort out her past and present issues. She had been nowhere near ready to accept this concept one year earlier, but now she agreed to this suggestion in an incredibly matter-of-fact manner. That's because she had thought intensely about her issues and had actually come to realize her need for psychotherapy on her own. That is always the best way, of course, but it doesn't need to happen that way. Gertrude was willing to take the first step to healing her mind, and one theory is that this approach would lead to the healing of her balance/panic and pain. This is not to say that her problems were primarily psychological. Indeed, the panic/balance and pain were occurring primarily as a result of physical disorders (nerves, muscles, ligaments, spinal cord, brain), but psychological factors certainly seemed to be driving the physical ones.

She had found a community fitness program for seniors but hadn't gone yet. Now she indicated she would surely sign up and participate three times a week in one-hour sessions.

She was ready to proceed, for an adventure, to change her life. It had taken a lot of soul searching and thought for her to get to this point. I congratulated her profusely on her amazing transformations and her decision to help herself. This was an example of the Finestonian dictum "It's never too late to get the help you need." Or, as the famous philosopher Rosa, my mother, said, "When you're dead, you're dead. Until then, you're not." And you can get help for anything as long as you show the will to do so.

Gertrude went for psychotherapy with a vengeance. She was a very determined woman, on a mission to heal her soul. She grew in mind and body. She continues to seek out new avenues for enlightenment. Now, several years later, her balance is much better, and she can walk on a sidewalk with her cane quite well. Her panic attacks are rare, but no, they haven't completely gone away. Complete resolution of all problems may be what we see in theatrical and movie performances. In real life we learn to manage, control, or lessen our bad habits, neuroses, and idiosyncrasies. And that's on a good day. Gertrude's mind and body are now talking to each other. The mind is respecting the body, and the body is acknowledging that the mind may have a role in its treatment. That's about as good as it gets.

CONCLUDING THOUGHTS

The accounts of Daphne, Tyra, and Gertrude are just a few examples of cases I have encountered in which childhood sexual or physical abuse seemed to be playing a major role in adulthood illness. Of course, I am not alone in establishing or recognizing that such a relationship exists. And it is not a simple path between abuse and pain. And every person's situation is different.

The scientific literature is replete with articles attempting to establish links between pain and a history of childhood or adult sexual, physical, or emotional abuse. Gastrointestinal symptoms, headaches, seizures, and diffuse kinds of body pain seem to be more prevalent in people (most study participants are women) with some history of abuse in their lives. Other investigators have tried to firmly establish the basis for this relationship, and there are a few studies that actually conclude that it doesn't even exist to begin with.

I can recount only what I see, what I read, what I feel, and, most important, what my patients tell me. Yes, there may be a few cases of "false memory disorder." A few years back, there was a lot of chatter about this entity: that people conveniently invent a history of childhood sexual abuse, supported and abetted and maybe even subconsciously or consciously "planted" by their psychotherapist, to explain away all of the emotional distress they are experiencing. The theory was that these patients were "using" a false memory of abuse to explain their maladaption to life, their sadness, unhappiness, or relationship problems. In general, these are not the types of people I am seeing. Usually, it's not a case of patients suddenly remembering their abuse—although that can happen—but, rather, the history of abuse rises to the surface of consciousness. Such patients know they were abused, but the abuse was not an event they wanted to share with anyone nor one they wanted to ponder on a continuous or daily basis—until now.

What seems to happen is that a new trauma, such as a motor vehicle accident, slip and fall, or sports injury, occurs and leads to physical injury and pain. The physical pain is an assault to the senses, just as the abuse was an assault. Sometimes the new trauma rekindles old memories, in some cases devastating ones. The edges blur, and the injured person experiences or relives the old trauma all over again, often, like Daphne, in the form of dreams. Dreams are usually not magical events that spring out of nowhere. They can be an expression of our innermost thoughts that are struggling to come out. I'm not a dream analyst, but my experience seems to point to the fact that violent dreams reflect some type of internal disturbance or conflict. The perpetrators of the violence in the dream may not be wholly representative of the patient's past encounters or experiences, but the dreams usually convey some psychic disturbance, some loss of equilibrium. Dreams are worth listening to, thinking about, analyzing, and putting into context.

Early on in my career, when I first recognized possible relationships between a history of abuse and adult pain, I took a somewhat "monosynaptic" approach. A synapse is the connection between two nerves, and, since nerves are everywhere, there are millions of synapses. My one-synapse or monosynaptic thought process focused on the physiological effects of physical, sexual, and emotional abuse. That is, I thought, a history of abuse initially leads to a state of chronic muscle tension, which the person simply copes with. It's not pain; it's a feeling of intermittent muscle tightness or tension. Then, when some sports injury or fall or fight-related trauma occurs, all hell breaks loose. The injured muscle and ligament structures show delayed healing, new stressors enter the picture to further delay recovery, and a persisting painful condition is the result. Breaking the cycle somewhere along the feedback loop of the pain condition (Figure 1.1 in Chapter 1) allows the body to sneak into itself and commence a healing process. This doesn't mean that an astute physiotherapist is not needed to get treatment and recovery going or that a medication to alleviate sleep disturbances or feelings of depression are not necessary. It does mean, however, that the healer and "healee"—the patient, client, or consumer—must be on the same page in recognizing the sometimes important role that dealing with a history of abuse may play in the patient's recovery.

Over the years, my interest in the effects of past abuse on the pain experience has broadened. Through my patients' sharing their experiences, I have become aware of other intriguing relationships between a history of abuse and pain:

- The experience of abuse leads not only to chronic muscle tension but to central nervous system (brain and spinal cord) changes, as well. The central pain receptor zones, the "way stations" that transmit pain from the periphery (hands, arms, feet, and legs), become more sensitive or too responsive or lack selectivity. With time, over years, a given pain stimulus is received differently in our brains, and pain becomes a constant companion. Fibromyalgia syndrome, discussed in Chapter 5, may be a partial product of this type of scenario.
- When you've been sexually, physically, or emotionally abused, your sleep may be chronically disturbed, and you are more prone to mood disorders such as depression, and therefore you are more distractible or less aware of your environment. As a result, you are more prone to accidents or mishaps that can lead to a musculoskeletal pain syndrome. It may be a car accident that occurs because your attention was a bit off, a trip over a branch that you just did not notice because your mind was on something else, a ski injury that wrenched your knee because your focus just wasn't on the bumps ahead of you . . . all are possible pain sequelae of the types of mind games that a history of abuse may play on anyone. This is not easy to prove, and it's not worthy of a Nobel prize, but I think these observations, considering but not *blaming* the affected individual, are worthwhile.
- A history of abuse seems to lead to more symptoms of pain, headaches, stomach pains, pelvic discomfort, and dyspareunia (painful intercourse). What do you do when you experience symptoms? You go to your doctor. He or she orders tests and, if the symptoms persist and the test results are negative or inconclusive, as they often are, then sends you to see other specialists. Specialists train very hard to master their specialty material. They want to help patients. In a study that colleagues and I published,[6] we found that women with a history of physical or sexual abuse were subjected to a significantly greater number of surgical procedures than nonabused women. Unfortunately, this was not surprising. One can see how surgeons, who so much want to help their patients, recommend the use of the tools that they are most familiar with: the scalpel, needle drivers, and sutures. Psychological and social factors may not be considered seriously as possible major contributors to muscle, pelvic, or gastrointestinal pain. Scars and repeated procedures or operations may be the result.

• The actual physical trauma sustained during cases of physical or sexual abuse (e.g., pelvic organs subjected to violent sex without lubrication, back and neck pain occurring as a result of being thrown, trampled on, or hit by a car) can lead to tissue injury that heals improperly or incompletely, leading to chronic persisting pain in the injured part of the body.

Many theories, many thoughts, much suffering. The most important quality that my patients and I strive for is hope—vitamin H. Without it, there is really nothing to ponder, nothing to live for. Buried among the initial presentation of pain, despair, addiction, and abuse is a flickering, barely perceptible flame that is hope. If the layers of callousness, past tragedies, family discord and violence can be peeled slowly away, the flame can begin to burn more intensely, until it is a roaring blaze.

To the abused—and you know who you are, and you have nothing to be ashamed about: You can find vitamin Hope and build a vital, strong body and mind around it. Your pain can diminish, one thought, one step, one barbell, one massage, one exercise, one counseling session, one lap, one acupuncture needle, one self-help group, one encouraging word at a time. To the rest of my readers: Understand and support what a person with a history of abuse may be going through.

NOTES

1. Community Safety Office, University of Toronto, http://www.communitysafety. utoronto.ca/assistance/abusive/abuseDefinition.htm (accessed October 12, 2008).

2. S. K. Burge, "How Do You Define Abuse?" (editorial), *Archives of Family Medicine* 7 (1998): 31–32.

3. H. M. Finestone, P. Stenn, F. Davies, C. Stalker, R. Fry, and J. Koumanis, "Chronic Pain and Health Care Utilization in Women with a History of Childhood Sexual Abuse," *Journal of Child Abuse and Neglect* 24, no. 4 (2000): 547–556.

4. R. A. Deyo, A. K. Diehl, and M. Rosenthal, "How Many Days of Bed Rest for Acute Low Back Pain? A Randomized Clinical Trial," *New England Journal of Medicine* 315, no. 17 (1986): 1064–1070.

5. H. M. Finestone, A. Alfeeli, and W. A. Fisher, "Stress-Induced Physiologic Changes as a Basis for the Biopsychosocial Model of Chronic Musculoskeletal Pain: A New Theory?," *Clinical Journal of Pain* 24, no. 9 (2008): 767–775.

6. Finestone et al., "Chronic Pain."

10

INSTANT RELIEF FROM MEDICATION, OR TREATMENT FOR THE MIND IS HARD TO FIND

He was tall, muscular, polite and soft spoken. The letter from the referring family physician read, "Back pain affecting his work. Please see and advise."

Kenneth was a former military officer whose job was to serve as a bodyguard for senior top-level executives. He walked in, sat down, and immediately said, "Doctor, I'm here because of my pain, I need to find some relief. Sometimes I have a hard time standing next to my boss's office door."

Whoa . . . I gently stopped Kenneth and explained what I was doing—that I was a physiatrist, that I tried to be a doctor who looked at the big picture, and I'd like to find out a little bit about him first. He sat back and relaxed—somewhat.

As with any job, doctors find that a certain thoroughness is necessary to get to the heart of the matter. We'd all like to miraculously diagnose the car's mechanical problem, fix the computer hard drive, or ascertain why our pricing is more expensive than our competitors', but we usually have to do our homework first—that is, listen to what the problem is. Look around. Medicine is no different. Yes, sometimes I can figure out within seconds that the swollen wrist I'm looking at is fractured. Pain issues, however, take time to understand and solve. And often there just aren't any shortcuts to get to the core of the matter.

Basic information was needed. Forty-one years old . . . two kids . . . married . . . recently moved from a larger city to assume his new job. He had a mild accent, from Africa, I thought, but his English was perfect.

I needed a medical history. Sometimes what happened in the past provides huge clues to what's going on, sometimes not. For example, one of the major predictors of back pain is previous back pain. Construction workers with a history of back pain are more likely to experience another episode of workplace-related back pain. Prostate cancer can spread to the back years after first developing. People with inflammatory bowel disease, such as Crohn's or ulcerative colitis, can also experience joint and back (especially in the sacroiliac, a big, tough joint that joins your pelvis to your sacrum, two major areas in the low back region) pain. Except for this current back pain episode, however, Kenneth hadn't noticed any back problems. As usual, I had to ensure that he hadn't ever contracted any infections or had any tumors or other relevant diseases. He had once had malaria but not recently.

He had been tested for the human immunodeficiency virus (HIV) as part of an application for a disability plan, and the test was negative.

HIV infection can present in many ways, and physicians must inquire about it for just about any group of symptoms, even though it is often uncomfortable to do so. Back pain with accompanying pain shooting down into the legs is possible in an HIV-infected person. I've had a patient who presented as a stroke survivor but who actually had toxoplasmosis of the brain, an infection common in people infected with HIV. Another presented with recurrent bouts of septicemia, or total body infection, a result of HIV's effect of weakening the body's immune system. Yet another first presented with generalized weakness caused by an attack on many of the body's nerves, a disease known as Guillain-Barré syndrome. An apparently celibate clergyman presented with blindness and dementia, also possible sequelae of infection with HIV. HIV and cancers related to the low immunity state of HIV-infected patients can attack just about any part of the neurological system. If physicians don't think about it, making the diagnosis can take a long time. Fortunately, with medical treatment, the disease can now be well controlled. But this is not the case in countries where treatment is not available.

Kenneth did not have HIV, and his pain was focused over the central part of his low back. It could spread—"radiate," in doctors' terms—to the upper part of his buttocks but never went further down his legs. This is a key point concerning a person's back pain. If the pain stays around the back and doesn't radiate below the level of the knees, one can generally assume that the problem is more related to the muscles, ligaments, or joints of the spine. In contrast, pain that radiates below the level of the knees into the feet often—but not always—means that a spinal nerve root is being compressed or affected. The nature of the pain is usually different as well, more burning or "electrical," more intense. A "pinched nerve" is the lay expression. A disc herniation (leakage of the jelly-like substance within the donut-like disc) can be the cause of radiating leg pain. In older people, "spinal stenosis," or a general crowding of the spine due to arthritis and "wear and tear," is the more likely cause of a compressed nerve.

These, however, are just "rules of thumb." If the pain travels only to the level of the ankle, the rules are not as clear. That's why we need doctors and other health professionals such as physiotherapists, chiropractors, and osteopaths to wade through these issues.

"Any other specific signs and symptoms, such as fever, chills, weakness, or loss of bowel or bladder function?" I asked. These are the dreaded "red flags" of back pain that lead one to suspect a more serious back problem. They imply an infection, tumor, or other disease, such as multiple sclerosis, which, although they are very uncommon causes of back pain, can happen. "No, doctor, none of those kinds of feelings," Kenneth responded. Good.

"Anything make the pain better?" As I have discussed in Chapter 2, it is important to ask questions about PQRSTU: the pain, its quality, radiation, severity, and timing, and under what circumstances. Questions about what makes the pain better and what makes it worse are also usually among the questions that doctors ask. If the pain is relieved really well by aspirin, it may mean that a rare but benign (not cancerous) tumor called osteoid osteoma is present. If the pain is made worse by activity, well, that's pretty common with most types of back pain. If the pain worsens and shoots down the leg when you cough, sneeze, or have a bowel movement, it may mean that a spinal nerve is being tickled or squeezed by a disc. So, "better or worse" questions help to focus in on the diagnosis.

"Tylenol [acetaminophen] makes the pain much better."

"Oh, when do you take this medicine and how many times a day?" I asked.

"What I do is I place a few tablets in my pocket so that I have them available to me at any time. I take two at a time about two to three times per day."

"How long does it take the medication to work?" I then inquired. Asking about medication use can elicit new medical information. People often don't think of certain medical illnesses that they may have until I ask them about their medication. For instance, when I ask a patient whether she has experienced any past medical problems, she may answer, "None." Then I find out she is taking thyroid replacement medication or antidepressants. Patients often do not consider their hypoactive (decreased performance) thyroid or depression to be a medical condition. I digress. I'm not really sure why I asked him how long it took for the medication to take effect. It is not a usual question, but it makes sense, as different medications have varied chemical properties, coatings, absorption profiles, and half-lives (how long it takes the drug to go from full to half-concentration in the bloodstream).

Kenneth told me that within seconds of placing the acetaminophen tablets in his mouth, the pain immediately disappeared—*instant pain relief.* This was a puzzling piece of information. Medication taken orally (by mouth) takes time to digest. It takes time for any medication to move from the mouth to the stomach and intestine. Then there is the drug's absorption into the bloodstream and subsequent travel to the brain or area around the injured part, that is, the knee, neck, great toe, or wherever. That's quite a journey. Assuming a healthy liver and kidneys, the primary body organs that handle any drugs we ingest, it takes about 30 minutes for pain medication to start working. But Kenneth's pills produced a pain-relieving effect as soon as he popped them into his mouth.

Hmm . . . I sensed a possible thickening of the plot. *What is going on here?* If it was not physically possible that the medication was providing him with relief, then what was relieving him of his discomforting pain?

I decided that I needed to acquire some background information. Time is always an issue in my medical practice, but almost invariably I find that information about a patient's childhood or adolescence can be important when discussing pain and probably any other medical health issue. Kenneth seemed a bit perplexed with this mode of questioning but agreed to continue.

"Where did you grow up?" He had grown up in an African country. "What was it like growing up as a child?" "Oh, it was a normal kind of life." I could see that Kenneth was a man of few words. It was time to venture into uncharted territory. Medical school and residency training could not take me there. Intuition, personal experience, past mentors, and the human condition would be my guides. Blind alleys and dead-end paths would be inevitable, but the journey needed to be made, or so I thought.

"What kind of family did you have?" "My mother was not around. She lived in another village. My father and his family raised me." "What kind of father was he?" "Oh, fine." Such short answers. Do I accept them and move on? Is it important to find out more about parental relationships when discussing a painful back? Yes, sometimes it is. So I continued.

"What do you mean? Was he a tough man, a soft man, did you get well taken care of, did you have enough to eat?" At the same time my mind was hurtling ahead to how he got to North America in the first place, what led him to become a bodyguard, and how he coped with his work and family life. *Slow down, Finestone. You can't figure out a person's entire life in one sitting.* I often have to remind myself about this important bit of information.

"My father was an alcoholic. He would drink a lot, so sometimes I would not see him for days, but my aunts and uncles took care of me in the village. We never had enough food to eat, but we managed." "Did you play with other kids?" "Oh, yes . . . we would play football on the hot ground. I had no shoes, and I remember how very hot my feet would become while running. We had no nets to kick into, and our ball was made of rags, but we had fun. . . ." So, no food, no shoes, no regular mom, an alcoholic dad, poverty as a child.

"Get along with your dad?" "He was mean when he got drunk and would beat me, but that didn't happen too often." No food, no shoes, no regular mom, very good village and family support, abusive dad when inebriated. . . . Who cares about this information? What does it have to do with pain or illness? Why was I asking these questions? Well, I do consider alcoholism in a parent to be a pain risk factor, a factor that enhances the possibility of developing future pain, as outlined in Chapter 6. But, overall, I was trying to understand what made this man tick. From there, maybe I could find out what was going on with this man emotionally and whether tension or other emotional factors had something to do with his pain.

Although his background and country of origin were very different from mine, I have found that this kind of gap is usually not an issue. The factors involved in tracking down pain origins, risk factors, and associations are similar worldwide. A tense, tough, hard, complex upbringing can lead to tense, hard, and complex muscles and ligaments and, subsequently, pain. Excessive muscle contraction, impaired blood flow, and immunological changes occurring as a result of psychic distress can develop. Changes to the spinal cord and the brain as a result of both chronic pain and mood states such as depression, have been described, as well. These were all possibilities to consider in Kenneth's case.

They are, of course, not always relevant, but that's what makes the digging even more interesting. And there was still more information to acquire.

Speaking about digging, my role as pain detective is therefore sometimes closer to that of a *pain archeologist*—digging and sifting through the sands of time. A shard pops up to the surface, and I have to decide whether it is part of a bigger vessel that can be reconstructed or just a useless piece of pottery/ information that goes in the archeological dig's garbage bucket at the end of the day.

I needed to move on—the waiting room had other clients—but the information provided by Kenneth thus far compelled me to ask more questions. "Wow, it seems like you've been through quite a lot in your life. It sounds like your childhood in Africa was quite a stressful time."

"Oh, no, Dr. Finestone. In my African country, we don't have stress." "What do you mean, you have no stress?" "We don't have such a word in our language. We don't know what stress means—that is a North American term—we just don't have it in our vocabulary. We do not need such a word." He seemed to be quite proud of this state of affairs.

Where to go from here? He had just described all kinds of childhood events that could have led to fear, worry, concern, and, yes . . . stress! He didn't seem to feel that stress was an issue, but he also didn't seem to appreciate what the term meant. And, although the background he described was a tough one, who is to say that it is any different from that of a million other like individuals? So he does not consider stress an issue. Do you have a problem with that, Dr. Finestone?

While I'm sitting right across from this gentleman, my mind is engaged in a further rapid internal dialogue happening in real time. Do I pursue this set of circumstances further? Push the issue? Somehow force him to acknowledge that, yes, he had stress but that he is not admitting to it? Maybe a few years back, I would have taken that tack, but there did not seem to be any point in pursuing that approach. At this point, the more I practice medicine, the more I realize that I have to let the patients tell *their* story. My hope that *they* will then listen to what *they* have just said comes next, but this does not have to happen right away.

I decided to simply mention that maybe Kenneth thought about stress in a different way and that perhaps we'd talk about this later. His brow wrinkled a bit—he seemed to be contemplating something—and we moved on. Finding out what Kenneth did in the course of a day's work and how he got there was next on the agenda.

It was a long journey from Africa to North America. He had immigrated to a large city in North America as a child, sponsored by a family member who had preceded him. His country was war-torn, and he was associated with the fighters for the wrong side. It was time to leave. I would have loved to obtain more information about these circumstances, but I did not.

In Canada, he completed high school and was then accepted into a college-based criminology program. He volunteered with the local police force and eventually moved into a special military police force.

Kenneth loved his work, and he was ambitious. He met a woman of African descent and married her while in his late twenties. Life was going very well. He was recruited to the worlds of industry and finance. His current job involved being the bodyguard of very senior executives who traveled frequently all over the world. He had to stand most of the day while wearing a uniform with a heavy gun belt attached.

Let us now wander back to the immediate pain-relieving effect of Kenneth's medication. Many therapeutic answers were plausible. The famous "placebo effect" immediately comes to mind. Can one's hoping or assuming that a medication will work enable an inert placebo, or "sugar pill," to produce a cascade of bodily and/or brain reactions that result in pain reduction? Although well known, the placebo effect is a poorly described entity. We're not sure why a placebo may be an effective treatment. Your doctor will not prescribe you sugar tablets while at the same time telling you that they contain powerful healing medications because it would not be ethical. A scientific medical study evaluating a new drug may, however, provide you with first a placebo and then the drug being tested. Then the effects of each treatment are compared. In many studies, the placebo has been found to be more effective than the drug. A placebo provides a benefit to a patient about 30 percent of the time. Studies rarely discuss how long the placebo's effect actually lasts, so all of this information is really not that helpful.

A doctor's reassuring and caring words, however, may be part of a placebo response, for example, a better recovery from an illness. This does not mean the patient had a bogus malady; rather, it may be just another manifestation of the intense relationships between the mind and the body. The placebo response simply indicates, once again, that happiness, confidence, mental stability, reassurance, and many other factors can combine to create potentially healthy body behaviors and reactions. No more, no less.

Was Kenneth's pain due to pressure on muscle groups, which immediately relaxed when he perceived that the pain medication would perform its magic? Was the pain not physical at all but a *brain pain*—a series of signals not related to any specific physical injury by which the brain indicates to the person *I am in pain . . . stop!* These are tough questions, but ones that are always worth discussing, in my opinion. Unfortunately, there are usually no immediate answers—just speculative thoughts.

The doctor or therapist that you are seeing may have specific ideas about the nature of your pain, which will affect his or her treatment approach. A chiropractor focuses on the spine's effects on body health, a physical therapist often focuses on posture, a massage therapist on the muscles and fascia. Anesthetists and interventional physiatrists focus on pain-relieving injections, and orthopedic surgeons may advocate surgery. This all makes it pretty hard for a patient in pain to understand all of the potentially disparate messages and treatment suggestions.

What is going on here? More questions. "How is your job going? Are there any parts of it—bending, lifting, or twisting—that cause your back pain to occur?"

Kenneth thought that his job was going well. He could not identify specific physical aspects of the job that caused specific back pain incidents. He did note, as back sufferers often do, that the back pain increased as his hours of standing accumulated and that prolonged sitting seemed to lead to more back pain than standing. Sitting applies more pressure to the low back discs than standing, and therefore Kenneth's symptoms made much sense.

Kenneth was very proud of his new position. His stature in his company and his salary had steadily improved over the past years. He was pleased that he could provide for his family and that his children were growing up in a healthy atmosphere.

At the risk of being annoying, I asked, "Are there any stresses that are affecting your new life—job, family. . . ?" "Well, my wife worries about me. She thinks I will be killed. Some mornings she begs me not to go to work. I must pull myself away from her arms. She also doesn't like living here at all and is not happy with our neighbors, but that's okay, we must manage." *Mama mia!* I was very concerned about these remarks. I imagined a *New Yorker* cartoon showing a suburban uniformed male leaving the front door of his home, with his wife attached to his wrists, somewhat like handcuffs, dragging her along the walkway while muttering, "Honey, I know you think my work is dangerous, but this is ridiculous."

Kenneth did not feel comfortable talking about worry and stress. Again, I felt a bit like a "nudnik," a term my grandmother used for an aggravating, bothersome person.

I proceeded to his back exam. First the doctor looks; nothing much to see. Sometimes I may note a hairy mole, which can be a sign that a spinal birth defect called spina bifida is present. Sometimes the person is shifted to the right or left, possibly indicating a spinal nerve root injury. Next is the evaluation of movement, or "range of motion." Kenneth had talked about having pain in his lower back, associated more with bending than with extending. The movement itself, however, was "within normal limits," doctor-speak for okay. All aboard for palpation, the application of the fingers to the flesh. Sometimes this is done before range of motion testing, but more often, to avoid causing pain that could then impede my assessment of the motion, I palpate first. I noted local tenderness when I pressed on the muscles that course alongside the spine, the paralumbar muscles. Definite physical findings were therefore evident, but at the same time they were fairly nonspecific. Normal neurological examination: normal reflexes, power, and sensation.

The diagnoses that I therefore had to consider included low back strain, low back sprain, mechanical low back pain, or lumbago (an old term, rarely used). These were not very specific terms. I pretty much could rule out a spinal nerve compression or bone tumor or generalized arthritic condition.

I left the room, and Kenneth removed his gown and put his uniform back on. We then talked about treatment. He had already been to physiotherapy and did not find that this produced any great changes. He ran two to three miles three to four times per week and experienced no or minimal pain while running. Structural damage to the spine due to arthritis or tumor or serious muscle injury would almost certainly have been painful under these conditions. More good news.

Ergonomics, the relationship between the work environment and the body, was discussed. Could some adjustments be made to his standing schedule? Could he have more opportunity to vary his sitting and standing? Could he find a lighter gun belt? Was the chair he usually sat on comfortable and supportive? Did he put a pillow in the area of the small of his back while flying in a jet plane to stabilize the spine's contour? These are all small but potentially important measures.

Kenneth and I then began to discuss the fact that the instant pain relief with acetaminophen didn't make a lot of sense in terms of the drug's action. Obviously, I had to tread carefully here. But it did make a lot of sense, however, for other reasons. The physical back pain was possibly being aggravated and even caused by stress, anxiety, and worry. These feelings can lead the paralumbar muscles to knot up and become tense. The thought of a healing pill produced pain relief by relaxing those muscles, improving the blood flow to them and allowing them to be more flexible. But then, because they were injured, they went back to their painful state within a few hours. These are simplified explanations, but, as described in Chapter 1, I think they make medical sense in the context of the current scientific literature. Kenneth listened and seemed to ponder my words. Like so many in our small world, he appeared to be very uncomfortable with these concepts.

So here we were: a hard-driving, successful, 41-year-old male of African descent; an alcoholic, sometimes abusive, father; poverty as a child; success as a bodyguard for the highest level of industry executive; a physically demanding job; and a wife who feared for his safety on a daily basis and sometimes didn't want him to leave the house to go to work. He felt that stress was not part of the vocabulary of his homeland but appeared to appreciate some of its negative effects.

As a doctor, one certainly does not want to *miss* a diagnosis, and this is usually the number one worry that we experience. Everyone has heard of a patient who was told it was stress and then died from ovarian cancer. Yes, that must have been stressful! It is frequently so much easier to just order a ton of medical tests, wait until they come back negative, and declare the patient well "except for your stress."

Kenneth didn't have much more to say. This led me to have a very heavy heart. When the patient cannot connect the dots after so much discussion, it is disappointing, but this was only a first encounter, and, realistically it likely had gone about as far as it could go.

After all, Kenneth was interested in getting better. I mentioned that I thought another next logical therapeutic step would be to refer him to a psychologist. This concept really upset him. Although he thought there could be benefits to seeing a psychologist and expressed his understanding of the possible connection between psychological and social factors and his back pain, the stigma attached to seeing a psychologist bothered him tremendously. It bothered him not only because of his cultural beliefs but, more important, because he worried that "if I go to a psychologist, maybe my supervisor will not think I'm up to the job. They'll think I can't cope . . . I won't be promoted . . . I can't do that!"

I called his family physician and discussed these issues. Kenneth's comments could not be discounted. I saw him a few more times. His pain would wax and wane, and he started to recognize more stress cues and their relationship to his pain. He was starting to notice, for example, that on days when his wife was particularly upset, he would experience worse pain. Reasoning with himself and talking to himself when he recognized such "pain triggers" helped sometimes to ward off a more intense pain episode.

But the reality of his situation prevailed. He had difficulty defining which life factors were important ones to consider. And when he did start recognizing some important issues, he couldn't understand why, if he just wanted to get better and ignored his psyche, he could not magically improve. While recognizing the important psychological and social factors that can make us physically and emotionally miserable is fundamental, it is unfortunately often only the first step in dealing with them. We then need to explore those emotions, those feelings of lack of self-worth, our tendency to be hard on ourselves, our perfectionism, our lifestyle choices. And, if we follow that kind of logic on our psychic journey, great things can happen, including vast improvements in pain and function. I have seen this occur many times.

I could not wholly reassure Kenneth about his fear that seeking psychological support could reduce his career potential. I did say that I thought his pain could be much better controlled and reduced if he received counseling.

In the end, he never received psychological help. He's still working as a bodyguard for top-level executives. The pain is up and down—some days very bad, other days much more tolerable. And society's acceptance of individuals' seeking psychological or social work counseling is still abysmal. We are going to have to incorporate mental health issues into everyday activity in general and medicine in particular. We need as a society to state that acceptance of the integration of mind-body issues in everyday schooling and in the workplace is as critical as paved roads, clean water, and electricity. It sounds a bit drastic, but understanding ourselves and others just a little bit better can lead to some powerful therapy.

For Kenneth, there was no eureka ending leading to lasting pain relief—just the ugly realities of life getting in the way. Kenneth was a bit farther ahead than he was when he first came in. He could talk to his wife a bit more about what he thought was going on in his body and his mind. His pain was less and under better control. That was good. That helped him. But his mission was far from complete. It would have helped if society were more accepting of psychological issues, but he couldn't change that situation. Maybe another year.

11

The Executive Asshole Syndrome, or Busy-People Arm-Pain Syndrome

The material for this chapter checked into my brain via a somewhat circuitous route. While I was passing by my hospital library, a book on display caught my eye: *The No Asshole Rule,* by Robert I. Sutton, Ph.D., a Stanford University professor. I borrowed it and found Dr. Sutton writing about mean-spirited individuals in the workplace who suck the life out of their workers and many who happen to cross their path. This bestseller emphasizes that these individuals can no longer be tolerated, and the author suggests many measures to root out and deal with the "assholes" in our workplace.

This chapter deals first with pain in the "asshole," our anal region, which some executives experience. Then I describe the typical musculoskeletal problems that executives and hard-driving, busy people in general may have. A few specific clinical scenarios have influenced me to appreciate how the mind and the body can work alongside each other effectively and destructively.

While working in a small hospital as a medical student, I was assigned to Dr. MacDonald, a general surgeon. Dr. MacDonald was a friendly, action-oriented surgeon, and the morning's schedule looked pretty busy: two hernia repairs, an ingrown toenail, and two "banding" operations to repair patients' hemorrhoids.

Although we hear commercials about painful hemorrhoids, most people don't know what they are. Even as a medical student, I had no idea how rubber bands were going to fix someone's painful bum.

My job was to help Dr. MacDonald in any way I could, and that included transferring patients from their rolling stretcher to the operating table if the porter or operating room staff wasn't immediately around to help.

As we were moving a groggy patient over, Dr. MacDonald muttered, "Another two cases of 'executive asshole syndrome.'" He was a blunt-speaking man with an occasionally salty tongue, so I was not too surprised to hear these words in the sanctity of the operating room. The hemorrhoid patient was then put to sleep by the anesthetist, or "gas passer," as these specialists are sometimes called, because they administer specialized gases by masks or tubes to render the patient incapable of feeling pain and the cutting, grinding and suturing that go on during a surgical operation. I now had the opportunity to ask Dr. MacDonald about the foreign-to-me term "executive asshole syndrome."

"Oh," Dr. MacDonald said, "it's a term I made up a few years ago for these particular guys. They are hard-driving businessmen, wearing nice suits, drinking too much booze with their cronies in the bar to calm themselves down, wolfing down their breakfasts and lunches so they can get back to work. They are always in a rush.

"So they wake up every morning, and they usually didn't have enough water to drink or fiber to eat the day before. Their main liquids were coffee and booze. They then really have to go, defecate. Instead of sauntering to the toilet and relaxing a few minutes, they are men on the move. Their mind is already on their morning appointments, and a little bit of sweat is accumulating under their armpits because they are worried about being late. Now they really have to make that dump. Instead of relaxing their anal sphincter, it's tight and their poop is hard. It's like trying to shove a brick down a constricted sausage. And, man, they try to push that brick through as fast as they can because they have people to see, bills to pay, competitors to stomp on. Pressure builds up from below, veins start bulging, and the rectum and anus are working overtime, squeezing their muscles as hard as they can. They then feel a ripping, tearing feeling down below. The brick drops, and they wipe themselves. They jump up in fright because of the pain of their new anal fissure and because of the fact that they're peering down at red drops of blood on the toilet tissue. The blood is courtesy of their anal fissure, a crack in the inner skin or mucosa of their anus, or some hemorrhoids—stretched-out, floppy, blood-filled vessels that, instead of staying inside, flop outward for the world to see. Get that, kid—that's the 'executive asshole syndrome.'"

Executive asshole syndrome made a lot of sense to me: the dehydrated, stressed, coffee-drenched, constipated, rushing businessperson who doesn't even have time to defecate properly. A fairly benign, take-it-for-granted process like pooping becomes a wicked series of events involving torn tissues and pain and/or bleeding from the rectum. The cycle continues because the anal fissure is painful, the person bears down even harder and avoids going to the bathroom to delay this defecation pain. Pressure mounts, which leads to a buildup of juicier hemorrhoids, and, voilà, a simple routine morning act becomes a "daymare."

Dr. MacDonald applied rubber bands tightly around the loose hemorrhoids or veins with the idea that they'd eventually dry up and die. The procedure, as far as I know, doesn't always work. With regard to the painful anal fissure, it's like a small tear that is symptomatic every once in a while. He would tell his patients to slow down, eat more fiber, and drink more water, and with time the fissure usually healed itself or at least stopped being painful. That's what I tell my patients.

Executive asshole syndrome. After I became a doctor of physical medicine and rehabilitation, I quickly realized that busy, hard-driving executives, office workers, and even factory workers got into a lot of musculoskeletal trouble, as well, while exhibiting some of the behaviors during their morning routine that Dr. MacDonald alluded to. So let's now move from the no-asshole rule and executive asshole syndrome to the caring, hardworking, sometimes slightly masochistic office-based people who can get into a "pile" of pain trouble.

Tom comes immediately to mind—49 years old, hair nicely coiffed, nails polished to a lustrous shine. I always notice fingernails, likely because my hard-bitten ones are in a constant state of forlornness. Sometimes I stop biting my nails and even go months leaving them alone. I become so proud of them. Then some stressful event happens or I'm preparing a talk or lecture, and bang! my nail-biting comes back again. Oh, well—as I tell my patients about quitting anything, from smoking to nail-biting to excessive eating, "the more times you show yourself you can refrain, the greater the chance that next time you really will be able to quit."

Tom was a branch bank manager, and he was really good at his job. He could schmooze with the best of them, and his success in obtaining blue-chip clients showed how well he performed.

But Tom was really hurting. You couldn't tell by looking at him, but he was hurting. When I asked him to describe "in one sentence" where his pain was, he stated, "my shoulder, my neck, my hand, my head, my back." Pretty quickly I concluded that (1) this was not going to be a short visit and (2) this was not going to be the last time I saw him.

Superficially, Tom looked like a healthy guy, but when I took his medical history it emerged that he had had more than his share of injuries or traumas. When he was 25, he injured his back. Pain was shooting down his leg, and he required back surgery to repair a ruptured, or "herniated," disc. As it often does, the surgery eliminated the leg pain, but he always experienced a "little bit" of low back pain, which he "lived with." He loved to mountain bike and once a year or so would get into a fairly serious accident. He cracked his left collarbone, or clavicle, on one occasion and dislocated his right shoulder another year. He always bounced back well, but he experienced a "little bit of stiffness" left over from the right shoulder injury and a "bit of aching," too.

Over the years he didn't make much of his pains—they were a nuisance, but that's about it. He coped with them and went on with his life.

Tom was always fairly glued to a computer but these days even more so. His right hand was melded with his mouse, as everything in the bank's operation was now mouse driven.

I am seeing more and more injuries that appear to be directly related to use of the computer mouse. Why? Well, nature didn't design the majority of our muscles to be working all the time. For instance, when you're just sitting quietly at your desk or on a chair, precious few muscles are being activated. The skeletal muscles, the chunky stuff in your arms and legs, are quiet at rest. When you decide to move a specific part, like your arm or leg, electricity passes through the limb, but only then. Our muscles were therefore more designed for "stop and start" activities. Even when we are engaged in a strenuous, prolonged task different muscles are constantly turning on and off.

But what kind of muscle activity is demanded when our hand is perched on top of the computer mouse, gripping it as if we were feeding it cheese all day? It's so hard to relax our hand and forearm when it's attached to a mouse all day—we have to apply just a little bit of constant tension to the mouse, and that's bad for our poor muscles because they just were not designed for that kind of prolonged action.

About two years earlier, Tom's mouse work increased somewhat. He started to notice "just a little bit" of aching in his right forearm extensor muscles—the muscles that extend, or bring up, the fingers rather than curl them into the hand. These are the "piano-playing" muscles: If you place the fingers of your left hand on the back of your right forearm just below the elbow and pretend you're playing the piano with the right hand, you will feel the rippling of these muscles.

A "little bit" of pain is tolerable, as we all know, but gradually Tom was noticing that the pain was becoming less and less tolerable. It was becoming a "grade 4" type of pain. In sports medicine, injuries are described as being part of a continuum. Grade 1 is transient pain, such as soreness occurring at least several hours after an injury. Grade 2 is longstanding pain of two to three weeks' duration that is typically present late in the particular physical activity or immediately after the activity. Grade 3 pain is usually present in the middle of the activity, progressively moving closer to the beginning of the activity. Grade 4, the most serious, is basically pain at rest and implies not just a breakdown of the soft tissues (muscles and ligaments) but a severe disturbance in the person's function.

Initially, Tom would notice pain starting on Thursday or Friday, after a long week of "mousing." The pain would usually let up over the weekend, and he would be "as good as new" by the time Monday came around. Now, however, the weekend was not enough to soothe his aching forearm muscles, and mouse work on Monday morning really bothered him. He was popping extra-strength Tylenol every three to four hours, but they didn't help much. Sleep was becoming disturbed because even placing his arm under his pillow bothered him—it was so hard to find any kind of comfortable position. And he needed his arms because there was "so much goddamn work to do."

Tom was also a weight lifter, an activity he had been doing since his youth. The weight room, then and now, sounded like his personal temple, his sanctuary. He would pop on his earphones, blast Black Sabbath into his eardrums, and pump the hours away.

But now his joy, weight lifting, was becoming a nasty, pain-inflicting enterprise. Certain machines were becoming impossible to perform on because of the severe forearm pain that they elicited. He exchanged 18-pound barbells for 8-pounders, but that did not do the trick. Really slowing down or refraining from weight lifting appeared to be—at this point—just about out of the question. It was part of his blood, guts, and DNA. If he couldn't lift weights, he just couldn't feel the same. And his previous dislocated shoulder was acting up, too.

It was time for Tom and me to regroup, take a deep breath, and start figuring out what was going on. His story was way too familiar to me, but a few more details were necessary.

Tingling or numbness in the hand? Carpal tunnel syndrome is a problem caused by pressure on one of the main nerves, the median nerve, which courses through the wrist. It leads to nighttime tingling of the hand, particularly the thumb, index, middle finger, and half of the ring finger. "Nope, I don't have that," said Tom. He also wasn't experiencing any problems peeing or pooping. I have to ask everyone this question even if there is only a remote chance of a spinal, neck, or back problem. Bladder and bowel incontinence are about the only problems that, if related to a spinal cord injury, require an *immediate* doctor visit. Tom was a bit constipated and occasionally experienced some pain with defecation. He probably had some parts of the executive asshole syndrome, but it did not seem that he had a spinal cord problem.

Tom was really hurting. Besides the deep aching forearm pain, he also described aggravating right-hand pain. There are many muscles located in the hand, which basically fill up all the gaps and spaces between the bones. In my experience, these hand muscles, the interossei, the lumbricals, and the muscles of the thenar eminence (area around the thumb) and the hypothenar eminence (area around the pinkie), become pain-causing structures. And why not? Doctors and therapists just don't think of them as they would a biceps or other larger muscles of the arm. We don't have too many names to describe pain coming from sore, injured small hand muscles. Sometimes heavy use of the thumb can result in a tendonitis problem called de Quervain's tenosynovitis, in which leather-like slips of tendons become inflamed as they move back and forth in the sheath that envelopes them. Pain at the base of the thumb and side of the forearm can result. Sometimes "crepitus," a crinkling, rough-paper type of sensation below the skin, can also happen. Tom didn't have this problem.

More often than not, mouse and keyboard users experience a nonspecific ache in the palm of the hand, often accompanied by a feeling of "numbness." Patients, including Tom, have said to me, "I can feel things with the hand; it just doesn't feel the same as my other hand." This situation seems to drive my neurology colleagues crazy. They like to see specific "deficits," or what the average person would call problems in feeling or sensation. A complete neurological sensory test includes testing for light touch (e.g., with a tissue), pinprick (e.g., with a disposable paperclip or device made expressly for this purpose), vibration sense (e.g., with a tuning fork) and proprioception, or the "is your toe up or down" test. Sometimes MDs and occupational therapists may add "two-point discrimination": seeing how close you can appreciate the simultaneous pressure of two probes on your fingertips. If we were getting really fancy, we might press a specially quantitated bendable nylon device called a Semmes–Weinstein monofilament to your skin to ascertain your sensory strengths and deficits. But enough digression. Tom's sensation was fine.

Tom just couldn't figure out why he was so sore and why his hand felt "weird" on an on-and-off basis. And his clinical situation was frustrating to him.

"I'm pretty young—why is this happening to me?" Excellent existential questions. I didn't have immediate answers. More information was needed.

I wanted to know more about the right shoulder pain, the "bit of aching" he experienced. "When did it start? Any specific day, or did it begin with a specific exercise?" He definitely felt a specific tearing sensation while weight lifting one particular afternoon. "What did you do then?" I asked. Sheepishly he answered, "Not much. I hung my arm to the side, and for the next few weeks I could barely use my arm it was so painful. I continued doing some bench pressing, but of course with less weight—yeah, I know that was dumb." Dumb, perhaps, but so common in males—ignoring their injuries even when they were being rubbed in their faces, practicing denial. Why does this seem to be more of a "male thing"? Could it be that men like to fix things themselves and are less likely to ask for help for any task? Society paints them as invincible, and, even if they don't feel invincible, males may feel compelled to at least act as if they are.

The shoulder and upper chest pain that he was experiencing actually had lessened with time and had become less problematic than what was currently bothering him most, his neck. *Your neck?* I thought. *Your neck? I don't want to deal with yet another part of your body. Enough parts are hurting already!* I hope my facial expression did not convey my inner shouting session. What initially seemed like a fairly straightforward situation—a bank manager with arm pain—now involved hand, forearm, and shoulder pain, and he had neck pain, to boot.

Now, I enjoy a complex problem, but you, the reader, must know that doctors, like anyone else, are usually happier when they are dealing with simple problems that they can deal with efficiently, thoroughly, and quickly. That's just the way life is—human beings are happier when they can get the job done in a manner that's not too uncomfortable. This case was rendering me uncomfortable. I felt that I could not be superficial. I needed to take out the medical detective shovel and start digging around. Tom's office environment seemed to be a good place to start.

Often I see office-related injuries that started for numerous reasons, such as:

- A nasty boss—perhaps an inhabitant of Dr. Sutton's *The No Asshole Rule* book—who makes the employees nervous, stressed, and overworked. Muscles and ligaments can bear the brunt of this assault.
- A fellow employee is on disability and no one is hired to replace him or her, so everyone has more work to do.
- A fellow employee who was on disability returns to work with physical restrictions and can't do all of the work that he or she used to do. The rest of the employees must pick up the slack and work harder, and this leads to new arm and neck injuries. Resentment lurks in the background, as well.
- The company is on shaky financial footing and is not hiring enough staff to cope with the workload. This contributes to overuse of multiple muscles, joints, nerves, and tendons. Pain and disability result.

"Anything special happening to you or your office or both?" A resigned, somewhat exasperated look appeared on Tom's face. "Well, yes. . . ." He then recounted that he was being actively recruited by a competitor bank, how he had essentially said yes, how already senior colleagues at work were treating him in a very mean-spirited manner and had tried every measure to delay or block his departure, and how he was counting the weeks until he could remove himself from this toxic environment.

Oh, I thought to myself. *This is a wonderful recipe to cook up neck pain if I ever saw one. One part overwork, one part preexisting injuries, two parts toxic-waste-dump office attitudes, three parts heavy mouse and keyboard use.* Nothing that I'd want to eat or drink, but that's what it was—a mess that needed some clean-up. At least that's what I thought. I could sort of see from the expression on Tom's face that he was a bit lost; he wasn't really clear why we were talking about work events and feelings in the first place. He didn't seem to be making any connections.

"How's all of this affecting the rest of your life, Tom—your wife, your kids, your own energy level, your mood?" Tom's body stiffened a bit, and he tapped his index finger to his head and said, "I think this is all getting to me up here, Doc. I'm tired all of the time. This past Sunday, my wife took the family to the movies, and I just could not go; I was bone tired. Even Father's Day, they all went out for dinner and I stayed home." Only Superman may be able to separate work life from home life, and even then Lois Lane figures out what's going on. Tom had three kids, two in high school and one in college, and a wife who was a teacher. They were not seeing Tom as often as they'd like. Sex was much less frequent—too painful, no time, and a decreased feeling of closeness prevailed. Sex often results from good times, free communication, and an ability to relax, and Tom hadn't been experiencing much of these over the past months.

So here was Tom, with "busy people arm pain" syndrome, hurting physically and psychically, not exactly recognizing how his stressful office situation might be exacerbating his musculoskeletal issues but getting there. He had pressure to perform in his usual office duties, and his new, stressful headhunting onslaught seemed to be really compounding his problems.

And that's what I see time and time again. A small muscle strain or tear becomes a larger one. A tolerable case of tendonitis gets angrier, redder, hotter, as a result of all the body chemicals, such as adrenaline, cortisol, substance P, and serotonin, that increase or decrease in response to change, stress, and distress. Tom was feeling all of these.

It was time for a thorough, detailed physical examination. There was a lot to look at. And that's often a problem. We doctors like to look at one part at a time. There are some family doctors who actually put a sign up in their waiting room, "One visit, one problem." Efficient, yes. Makes sense, sure. But obviously one cannot follow this rule all of the time. One can see, however, how being the doctor of a person with multiple needs, symptoms, and complaints can be quite difficult and exhausting. But that's a doctor's life.

I always have to ensure that the patient is not suffering from other specific diseases. Besides the specific muscle strain or overuse, most doctors carry in their brain some type of mnemonic or check list of diseases. Mine harkens back to my McGill University medical school days: KITTEN DIV—congenital (**K**), infectious, toxic, traumatic, endocrine, neoplastic, developmental, inflammatory, and vascular. For each of these categories, there are specific questions and physical examinations that help me to rule in or out a particular disease or syndrome.

Tom did not seem to be complaining of a rheumatological or joint problem, and his hands, wrists, knees, hips, and feet did not show any redness, swelling, or warmth (which would indicate inflammation). He was not losing weight or experiencing fever or chills, as one sometimes sees in a patient with cancer (neoplastic) or an infectious process. His blood tests were all normal. Thank goodness, other diseases besides the musculoskeletal ones discussed were not evident.

I proceeded to the musculoskeletal examination, the part of the physical examination that looks at the person's muscles, ligaments, and joints. First came inspection, palpation, range of motion—simplified by a well-known English orthopedic surgeon into "Look, feel, move." Tom's neck looked fine. When I pressed, or "palpated," his neck muscles, they were tender, as were the muscles just below, the trapezeii. He moved his neck rather slowly, but his movement, or "range of motion," was quite sound. He noted a little bit of pain at the end of the range in all the directions that the neck moves: forward (flexion, chin touching chest), backward (extension, looking up toward the ceiling), over each shoulder (rotation), and to the side (lateral flexion, trying to touch your ear to your shoulder). Range of motion sometimes, but not always, correlates with neck pain, that is, the greater the loss of range of motion, the more pain you have.

Examination of Tom's right shoulder showed really impaired range of motion. I was surprised. He could barely bring his right hand across his chest to touch his left shoulder. Now, that's stiff. Tom said that this limitation had been with him for years, ever since the "way back when" bike accident. He didn't even really notice it. The stiffness meant to me that he had less reserve and that doing an activity like weight lifting could rip or tear something more easily than if his shoulder had normal range of motion. Otherwise, there was some pain with motion, but not much. Tests looking for tendonitis or injury to the rotator cuff (so-called impingement tests) were normal. Overall, Tom's shoulder didn't seem to have anything really bad wrong with it.

Tenderness was noted over the fleshy forearm extensor muscles, the extensor digitorum brevis and longus and the extensor carpi radialis. There was pretty exquisite tenderness. I could elicit pain in them by having Tom bring his wrist upward while I was pushing down on it. This is called "resisted" range of motion. Pain occurs with resisted wrist motion if there is a muscle or tendon problem such as a tear or inflammation. No tenderness was noted over the outer bony part of the elbow ("lateral epicondyle"). This is where "tennis elbow," or lateral epicondylitis, is a problem (discussed in Chapter 4).

Fortunately, he didn't have it. His hand looked normal. There were no red-hot or swollen joints. He could easily make a fist, which further indicated that the finger joints were not stiffening up.

But when I palpated the muscles between the bones in the palm of his hand, the metacarpals, Tom felt much soreness and tenderness. The first dorsal interosseus, a slip of muscle between the thumb and index finger, was also tender. As is frequently the case, Tom was hardly aware of the actual degree of tenderness; he had become so used to feeling hand discomfort that his brain tried to kick it way in the back, into the outer recesses of the mind's gray matter. But the pain was still there, lurking, aggravating, and likely affecting his ability to deal with the slings and arrows of life.

A review of past medical imaging tests didn't really help much and actually contributed to some confusion—that can happen. Certainly, x-rays, MRIs (magnetic resonance imaging), and nuclear medicine tests—the "big three" when discussing imaging tests for muscles, ligaments, and joints, as well as for neck and back problems—have revolutionized how doctors think about their patients' musculoskeletal complaints. Not only can we now obtain wonderful, accurate images of a broken bone, as we may see from a standard x-ray, but we can better appreciate swelling or bleeding into a muscle or joint. We can discover, from a CAT (computed axial tomography) scan or an MRI, how the disc between two vertebrae (the building blocks of the spine) is herniated or spilling its inner contents outward and pushing on a nerve in its path. We can also gaze at fuzzy but helpful bone scan pictures that tell us, by way of a little dark spot, that something is wrong in one part of the skeleton. Excellent. Much appreciated. Practice changing.

There's always a but. The "but" here is that sometimes the medical imaging tests that we doctors order lead to ongoing grief and confusion, as I've alluded to in a few other chapters. The best line I've heard from a medical colleague and that I use on a regular basis is this: "We treat people, not their test results." Although an MRI recently helped me diagnose a rare peripheral nerve tumor in the hand of one of my patients, the report on Tom's MRI of his shoulder was not helping us to better understand his health problems. The report stated that there was an abnormality in the area corresponding to the inferior (lower) labrum, or lip, of part of the shoulder joint. The million-dollar question was "What does this abnormality have to do with Tom's shoulder pain?" Very thoughtful question. Superior, or upper, labral tears, or "SLAP" lesions, do have some meaning and may be amenable to surgical repair. Inferior lesions—not substandard ones, but lower ones—are not surgically correctible, and the finding in itself is not indicative of a particular disease or orthopedic problem.

Fortunately, Tom did visit an orthopedic surgeon, who reassured him that the MRI finding was likely a longstanding problem related to his past biking injury and that surgery was definitely not recommended. If Tom had visited another orthopedic surgeon, the outcome might have been different. There is a state of the art, but it may not be as consistent as one would hope.

Because shoulder problems and the imaging of them are not part of a perfect science, the message here is that an abnormal MRI is not the final word on someone's pain. The imaging is an extension of the history and the physical examination—no more, no less. Sometimes, amazing new information may be obtained from the CAT scan or MRI or bone scan, but more often the test confirms what the doctor suspects. Tom's MRI report was not normal, but, in view of his symptoms, his actions, his past injury, and his physical exam, it was unlikely that the labrum problem was responsible for his shoulder pain.

Unfortunately, imaging tests for sore muscles are not completely state of the art. You may be experiencing a deep throbbing pain in your low back or buttock, but there are no adequate tests that show the depth of your suffering. Those beautiful charts of muscles that hang in my office are drawn by an artist—the depth of detail is portrayed by brush strokes. MRIs, CAT scans, and plain X-rays can't display the beauty of a work of art or the source of the pain. What's the message? The MRI may show a torn or frayed rotator cuff tendon or a ratty-looking tennis elbow. And that information may be very helpful. But it doesn't mean that that is the whole problem or that it is a problem that needs to be fixed surgically.

Other imaging tests that Tom had did not point to anything serious. His neck x-ray didn't show any arthritis except for a few "scattered degenerative changes" at multiple levels. I call that a "McDonald's coffee" sign, that is, with this x-ray finding and $1.25 you can buy a cup of coffee. As I've said, x-ray changes of a neck may be like wrinkles on a face: one doesn't like them, but they're not necessarily damaging or causing any problems.

Tom's neck pain seemed more muscular in nature: burning, aching, relieved by a warm shower or a neck rub. And his life circumstances certainly seemed to be causing or at least worsening his situation. His ability to cope with all of the dissonance and conflict in his life seemed to be both coming to a head and going to his head. Sort of a coming-and-going kind of problem.

Tom's neurological examination, consisting of motor (strength), sensory (feeling), and reflex components, was fine. No brain, spinal cord, or nerves seemed to be injured enough to cause the pain that he was experiencing.

Where to start? With the pain explanation and treatment diagram (see Appendix). We had some work to do. I called Tom over to sit next to me while we filled out the diagram together. It's much better if the patient and I can put our minds together to figure out both the diagnosis and the treatment. I have found that the more engaged the doctor and patient are in pursuing and solving the pain-related issues, the greater the chances of success and recovery.

We started on the diagnoses section. By taking into account the history, physical examination, and laboratory investigations (e.g., imaging test results and blood tests, which I was lucky enough to have received in advance), I thought we could come to some initial conclusions. This is a crucial first step because any treatment depends on an accurate diagnosis. Someone might just label Tom as having "chronic pain." That's not a diagnosis, but one hears it all the time. Usually the term means "there's a pain, it's lasting a helluva long time, there doesn't appear to be any immediate end in sight, and mood, feelings, vocational issues, marital problems, sleep difficulties, and myriad other issues have burrowed their way into the mix, like termites in a post. And the post is supposed to be holding your ceiling up." Maybe I should actually use these terms when I am speaking to my patients rather than just thinking them.

It takes scientists years to develop theories, teachers take days to months to create lesson plans, and lawyers often need months to build up their cases. But doctors usually must come up with a diagnosis in seconds, minutes, or hours. Of course, that is not always the case, and the investigation of a problem can take some time, like it is sometimes conveyed in an episode of the television program *House*. But quick assessment and diagnosis is the nature of medicine. The way medical problems often present quickly and the way doctors get paid (by the act) often contribute to the need to think, perform, and document quickly. And that's the way it is. I offer no solutions at this time, just food for thought. Especially since we're in the middle of Tom's particular case.

Tom's list of diagnoses was as follows:

- Forearm pain: musculoligamentous pain, meaning pain coming from the muscles and ligaments of Tom's mouse-using forearm. A synonym, I explained, would be myofascial pain. Particular muscles that seemed to be involved were the extensor carpi radialis longus and brevis and others in the vicinity. We didn't have to go overboard with the particular names. Tennis elbow didn't appear to be the problem, and neither did a specific nerve or bone injury.
- Hand pain: yup, pain in the muscles or ligaments of the hand. Not carpal tunnel syndrome. Interossei and lumbrical myofascial pain (names of some hand muscles) was a relevant diagnosis.
- Shoulder pain: this situation seemed a bit more complicated. An old biking injury. A history of weight lifting. Very limited range of motion on the physical exam, but no signs of a rotator cuff problem. An MRI that was abnormal but questionable as to what it meant. An orthopedic surgery colleague I later contacted confirmed my thoughts, which I conveyed to Tom. The MRI finding was likely insignificant, the shoulder pain was likely the result of a torn or injured structure, such as the shoulder capsule, a thin filmy layer of tissue that could not be imaged. Surgery: not a good idea.
- Last, neck pain: once again, muscle ligament pain with a smidgen of some "mild arthritis" thrown in for good measure. A nerve injury to the major nerves or nerve roots leaving the neck, or radiculopathy (radicle = root in Latin), was not evident.

Next, we discussed treatment. I made the usual Finestone comment: "A muscle ligament transplant should solve the problem: Take out the bad parts, get new ones, plug them in, and away you go." Tom pretty quickly recognized the facetiousness of my remarks, and I rapidly noted, "But of course we can't do that. So let's look at various factors and issues that can aggravate, improve, or screw up your injured muscles."

Habits such as smoking, eating to excess, and alcohol overuse were discussed. Alcohol was becoming a fairly regular dinner and after-dinner activity for Tom, at home and at bank-related meetings. Alcohol overuse is a possible sign of general dysfunction, and alcohol is a possible neurotoxin, as well. Can I say for sure that alcoholics have longer healing times than nonimbibers? I can't, but I think it is possible. Are you more likely to get injured owing to clumsiness, lack of attention, or imbalance if you're tipsy? I certainly do think so. Tom would consider how much alcohol he was transferring down his gullet.

Proper eating at regular times was briefly discussed. Tom was constipated, and some mornings were worse than others in this regard. To feel better and avoid executive asshole syndrome-type symptoms, I recommended drinking eight glasses of water a day, eating whole wheat bread, and maybe taking a tablespoon of psyllium daily. The latter is a natural algae product available in granular form in pharmacies and grocery stores.

On to sleep issues. His doctor friend had provided him with a medication like amitriptyline, an antidepressant that is used mainly for sleep disorders, headache, and pain (discussed in previous chapters). It had a great name like Elasteril (that's not the name), conveying that you'll feel more elastic or flexible. Actually, it made Tom sleepy. He slept better, and that was great. It didn't change his pain per se, but if you feel more rested, you can deal with any situation a little bit better—that's how I see it and explain it to my patients. There may be somewhat more complexity to the issue, such as improving the brain's sleep waves (as discussed in Chapter 5), but that didn't matter much to Tom or to me. Results were key, and better sleep was what we were after.

Exercise was discussed. Too much, too little? Tom had a combination of too much and too little. Too much weight lifting, which exceeded his pain tolerance as well as his shoulder range of motion. He needed to cool down his routine, not necessarily give it up altogether. He was willing to do this. I asked him to see the gym's trainer and discuss his routine with her. Trainers often have wonderful suggestions, but they need to know their limits and their clients' restrictions. I told Tom that he could move his shoulder into most positions but not if he felt his shoulder was ripping apart while doing the exercise. He also had to recognize that if his shoulder was so stiff so many years after an accident, he had to accept some limitation. This was not easy for him to do, as conveyed by his sighing and glum facial expression.

Next, we looked at ergonomics—the machine-body interface, an important issue in "busy people/office arm pain" syndrome and in every walk of life. There are too many devices thrown out on the market with breakneck speed that aren't thought out enough—car radio controls that are too small to handle, containers and plastic wrapping that are impossible to open, phone handles that need to be gripped, sometimes, as in Tom's case, for hours.

Tom had already thought about the phone issue. He asked about a wireless headset. As a bank manager, he had frequent phone meetings, and the speaker phone just sounded too "tinny." How about a headset that would enable him to walk around the room while talking or at least to move freely around in his chair without needing to use his hands at all? This certainly made a lot of sense to me.

I immediately wrote out a note for Tom to take to the workplace. I find this to be a very quick and effective way to deal with simple office ergonomic issues. You can always ask your doctor to do the same. Rather than type out a letter, boom, I write out the message "Diagnosis: office-related arm strain; needs telephone headset and office ergonomic assessment." The patient takes this to her employer, and often—not always—the purchases are made or the service ordered. Since the health insurance plans of provinces and states rarely cover an ergonomic assessment, a private company or individual usually must be engaged. Some proactive companies may have an in-house ergonomist who is ready for action, but that's not very common, in my experience.

Changing the mouse to the left hand or at least alternating hands was the next step. This can be a very significant step, and it really works. I told Tom that it would take some time to get used to, about three to four weeks, but with persistence he could become very adept at left-hand mousing. It seems simple, but so many people just don't think of this "shift to the left." Maybe their political persuasions wouldn't allow them to make such a change. . . .

One group that finds it very hard to shift the mouse to the nondominant hand are those who work in design, such as graphic artists and engineers who do a lot of computer-aided design (CAD). Even in these groups, however, I've seen it done. The main goal is to lessen the load on those aching forearm and hand muscles that are no longer on the plains and steppes hunting wild game. The modern office hunting ground is far more static and repetitive. You may have heard the terms "repetitive strain injury" (or syndrome) and "cumulative trauma disorder"—the arm strains and sprains, the tennis elbows, the de Quervain's tenosynovitis that occur with repetitive office work. Some doctors dislike these terms because they are neither specific nor indicative of a specific diagnosis. I agree with these points but still feel that the terms are valid and important. In the past, repetitive strain injury got a lot of bad press, particularly in Australia, where it was implied that people were somehow making their symptoms up. When the diagnosis was disallowed as a basis for disability payments, the number of claims rapidly declined. To me this means only that when you're not allowing complaints about something or at least not paying for them, fewer complaints related to that problem will be filed. It certainly does not mean that people don't experience sometimes disabling pain from performance of repetitive office activities, because they do. Definitely.

Tom felt that he could move the mouse to his left hand and said he would certainly purchase a telephone headset, he hoped with bank funds. He would wait until he moved over to his new job to avoid rubbing salt into already festering wounds.

Our shoveling in the psychological and social heap had already dug up a number of issues that could potentially have an impact on Tom's healing, recovery from injury, and the experience of pain, peripherally or centrally. We reviewed factors such as (1) worry, (2) anxiety, stress, and distress, (3) depression, (4) job disruption, (5) overwork, (6) child sexual or physical abuse and (7) alcoholism in family members or in the patient. I explained how this all worked, talking about some of the issues noted in Chapter 1. I outlined how increased stress in particular causes muscles to contract more and leads to varying combinations of poor oxygenation, biochemical changes, impaired immune function, and, ultimately, delayed recovery from injury.

Take these stress-related physiological changes, add various office and computer/mouse-related muscle, tendon and ligament injuries, and throw in the new stresses of a new job and angry work colleagues. Then finish off with the *effects* of chronic pain and stress, which included poor sleep, lack of energy, possibly depression, diminished sexual drive, change in roles as a husband and father, potential personality changes, and diminished concentration. It just goes on and on, and the result is a tired, stressed-out, exasperated bank manager who is in physical pain.

Tom's puzzled look relaxed a bit. He looked like he had been struck by something hard. "We're not going to solve all of the world's or your problems now, but we can take a few small steps. You have some thinking to do about how you fit into all of this stuff we've been talking about. I'm not a preacher or a psychologist, but you need to look a little deeper into your soul and help yourself figure out what's going on here. You are going to tell me, not the other way around."

I thought that a referral to a psychologist made a lot of sense; Tom didn't want to hear about this. Despite his psychological issues, he didn't think a mental health referral was necessary. He was very uncomfortable even discussing the issue. I respected that.

Keep exercising. Don't kill yourself. Drink less alcohol, work on the constipation, move the mouse to the left, get a headset, and get a life. Think about a psychologist. May be this was a bit too much for the first session, a bit too intense. But Tom's situation was getting quite serious and thus called for serious actions.

I had to sort of push Tom out the door. Despite my best intentions and although I had spent more time with him than I thought I could afford to spend, I still had to assume that classic doctor pose—standing by the door, hand on the doorknob, door ajar, patient still sitting, with facial expression pleading to the doctor not to leave. Why Norman Rockwell didn't paint that particular scene—it's far more common than a kid with his pants down—is one of life's major mysteries. Rockwell had more idyllic visions in his head when he painted his famous portrait of the doctor, I guess.

"We'll see you in two to three months," I said.

Tom returned in 11 weeks. The move to the new bank had gone extremely smoothly. His new employers were very supportive. They rapidly bought him a telephone headset. Many of his former clients walked across the street to do business with his new institution. There were the usual adjustments to a new environment, but nothing major. Tom felt wanted. There were fewer lines on his face.

He had moved the mouse to his left hand. This was definitely hard to do, but with time he got used to it. For the most complex tasks such as detailed spreadsheets, he would move it back over to the right, but not frequently.

The tightness and the soreness of the forearm were receding. It was definitely still there, but it was not keeping him awake at night. His hand could make its way under the pillow without his wincing. The neck pain was virtually nonexistent, but every two weeks, particularly if there was increased business in the office, pain would reappear.

Tom had laid off most weight lifting that involved the shoulder, and so the shoulder was much better, as well. He was still massaging the right hand with his left quite frequently—it had become a bit of a habit.

The head was a bit clearer, too. Tom now made reference to some very intense feelings that he had been having for at least six to eight months—feelings of sadness, negativity, a sense of being down in the dumps, that nothing was good. He hadn't talked about these emotions to anybody, including his wife or family doctor. Another "manly" act. It is not unusual for me to ask about "suicidal ideation," or thoughts of suicide. If a doctor is at all suspicious of depression, he or she must ask questions regarding suicide. Tom's jovial "up" manner apparently had been concealing some pretty heavy thoughts about possibly harming himself. The stress and tension he had been experiencing were that bad, and he could mention it only now.

Fortunately, these thoughts were no longer present at all. He felt somewhat hopeful about the future. As staff on the Stroke Rehabilitation Unit of my hospital often say, "There's no better mood treatment than getting better." If my patient recovers from the stroke, mood decline usually lifts, even without antidepressant medication.

But Tom needed to be watched. It seemed that he was out of the deep woods, but he was definitely not into a complete clearing, and I told him so. "Yeah, you think so?" he said somewhat quizzically. I could sense that he knew this was true, that his mood was still fragile, and care needed to be exercised.

I had actually contacted a psychiatrist and discussed Tom's case over the phone. The psychiatrist immediately picked up on the hard-working, driving intensity that I described: "What's driving him? That may be important." I told that to Tom, but he didn't want to pursue a referral to a psychiatrist. He had made so many positive gains that I did not pursue this further, for now.

Tom also related that he was slowing down. He tried to get home for more suppers, and family life was fitting into his agenda more.

The physical exam was improved. There was still tenderness with pressure over the forearm muscles and over the neck muscles. He was surprised about this latter tenderness because the experience of neck pain had diminished so much. This is a very common scenario: massage therapists, chiropractors, and doctors all find tenderness in muscles that the patient doesn't necessarily note on a regular basis. We don't always think of our pain on a second-to-second, minute-to-minute basis. But frequently the muscles are still harboring a little soreness or irritation that can be discovered by the clinician's fingers.

I told Tom that, overall, one could not expect a better result than what he had described. He was experiencing less pain. Specific body parts were less symptomatic. Instead of focusing on the deficits, I discussed why his improvements had likely occurred. This is a good exercise for all of us. Try to figure out "what went right," rather than the usual "what went wrong." Figuring out what positive things you did to achieve success may allow you to it more often and to take other, similar steps. Together we made a list of the various positive events that had occurred over the past months that had allowed Tom to improve his painful situation:

- His new workplace was welcoming and not confrontational, which contributed to quieting down the muscle activity; there was less adrenaline and fewer other stress-related biochemicals circulating in his system.
- He was not "trashing" his shoulder by repetitively forcing certain weights on it. He was controlling the forces induced about his shoulder, and pain relief was a result.
- He had made specific ergonomic adjustments: changed the mouse from Republican to Democrat, used a telephone headset to lessen gripping, and overall reduced right-arm trauma, giving injured muscles a chance to replenish and recover.
- Sleep was improved, and depression, which he almost certainly had, was lifted or lifting.
- He was more engaged in life, leading to better body awareness and better control of the types of things he ingested into his body, such as alcohol. This was leading to greater satisfaction. With all of these, he had reduced his pain for the most part.

This was a follow-up visit, and the time allotted was only 30 minutes, compared to the 60+ minutes of the first visit. I congratulated Tom on his improvement. He knew that he still had work to do. I again raised the flag of a mental health professional. Too bad there is such a stigma about getting psychologically healthy. Tom was not exactly wrong when he stated that he was concerned that visits to a mental health professional would "get on my record." Indeed, from what I have heard, even discussing mental illness, however mild, may affect a person's chances of promotion. Very sad. The people who try to get help for themselves and who will likely become more proficient and energetic employees as a result are in effect punished. But that's the current world we live in, and I have to accept that as a physician.

"Tom, I'll see you in two months. Keep thinking. Respect your mind and body. They are all you have."

Tom's third visit was more eventful. "No pain" in the right shoulder or "99 percent gone," without any new therapy initiative, witch doctor, or spiritual adviser. Hand pain virtually gone, too. Smiling.

He had been up until about 3 A.M. the previous night discussing bank policy. His expertise was being utilized! He found this exhilarating, but now he was quite exhausted. And he noticed that nagging, sometimes dagger-like jabs would start in his neck muscles under these types of circumstances.

We talked about the "drift" that any recovering workaholic, alcoholic, or intense person experiences at some point after a significant positive life change is made, that slow drift back to where we were before we became ill, that little voice in the back of our heads that tells us "we did it, we're fine now, we don't need to drink less or work less, we can now go back to where we were before." Maybe the little voice is a jaded Freudian "superego." Maybe it's the voice of denial that does not allow us to realize how serious our situation has become. We slowly, sometimes imperceptibly drift back to our dysfunctional ways. It's so sad when it happens. Like when a famous singer or movie star, like Amy Winehouse or Robert Downey Jr., falls back off the wagon. And I told this to Tom. I told him that I sensed a possible return to old habits. The Superman suit in the closet was possibly going to the dry cleaner's so that it could be ready for next week's or next month's bank activities. "You think so?" Tom asked. "Yes, Tom, I do. All your good work will quickly go down the drain. This need to hold back, to plan leisure activities, to plan family time, and to be vigilant about how much office work is to be done will *never* stop. And when you do stop doing those healthy checks, you'll start sliding and drifting and gasping. And you won't be good for anyone." Sometimes I have to be really blunt. If not, the message is filtered and I see it being chopped and cut up as soon as it's leaving my lips. Creating a bit of a fear of God, a scare, a shaking up. That was one of my thousand roles. Tom needed to know the consequences of his actions. I needed to contribute to the shake-up. He was salvageable, but, as I said, it's a lifelong journey to keep the demons at bay, to lead a life that is not harmful to mind, body, and soul.

Tom had come a long way. The primary issues were his musculoskeletal pain problems. They were what caused his intense suffering and drove him into my office. The solutions to solving these muscle, ligament, and tendon injuries involved multiple actions. Unfortunately, we all don't have control over our feelings, our environment, our family, our friends, our workplace. . . . The key message is that the injured forearm, shoulder, or hand, if approached at the right time, has the potential to heal. The human being, with his or her therapist, doctor, or other practitioner, must try to create the optimal environment in which those injured tissues can heal.

A toppled, broken bridge will remain that way. It will not repair itself. The human body, however, is a unique structure. It can heal itself by pouring more blood into the area, removing debris, laying down healthy tissue, creating a strong scar. But the tissue needs the right environment. Think of a seed in the ground. It can be the most expensive seed from the fanciest company around, but without good soil, watering, and fertilizer, the seed will just not perform. It will not sprout into a luscious, leafy green vegetable.

Tom's injured body parts needed to be physically, ergonomically, and spiritually nourished. Good things such as a headset needed to be added, and bad things such as overwork and mouse overuse needed to be taken away.

Are these such hard concepts to understand? Do we need to label all persisting pain as "chronic pain," pain that cannot be lessened, pain that we simply have to "learn to live with"? No. Of course, different pains require different approaches, but usually an inroad, a brief or long line of attack, or a flash of therapeutic light can be initiated to change chronic into sometimes or never.

The executives' assholes developed a syndrome because the executives rushed around and displayed no respect for body functions. But Tom's busy-people arm-pain syndrome was receding into the past. Tom was showing more respect for his body, and it was paying off in spades. By looking at sleep, exercise, ergonomics, weight, bad and good habits, and the role of physical and emotional stressors in his life, Tom was blooming, like a flower in the bank's office garden. He still had some work to do, but who doesn't? His muscles and ligaments recognized the lifestyle improvements, but they also sensed the improved blood flow, flexibility, and immune system effects. The mind and the body were working together, creating more than the sum of their parts.

I wished Tom well and told him I would see him in five to six months.

12

WRAPPING UP: PAIN, DISABILITY, SOCIETY, AND THE INDIVIDUAL

And now it is time to say goodbye. It is time to wrap up *The Pain Detective's* stories and summarize some of the principles and lessons learned. In doing so, I will offer new ideas about how society can change the way pain is dealt with, via the education it provides and the medicine it delivers.

A common thread that runs through the book's chapters is the need for individuals to recognize which physical, psychological, and social factors are playing a role in their pain problems. Ann "figured out" that a nasty, angry boyfriend was causing her back muscles to tense up and that this factor likely played a greater role in her pain than the underlying spinal defect, spondylolysis, that she had always had. Mandy, who worked in an armed forces special unit, experienced fatigue and pain. She came to realize that what happens in her life could affect her body, how mothering a mother may be one stimulus that influences the experiences of chronic fatigue.

Sally and Sam appreciated how being the child of an alcoholic parent can affect the way one carries one's body later on in life. Self-esteem and personal-worth issues can lead to excessive muscle tension, which, when combined with injuries, poor posture, and badly designed work stations, may result in pain.

Pain risk factors—all those issues relating to family, neglect, health behaviors and our physical, social, and psychological status that may contribute to a state of persisting pain—are a cornerstone of this book. They include smoking, too much alcohol, obesity, lack of sleep, poor work or home ergonomics, and lack of exercise or the right type of exercise. Stress, anger, financial problems, a history of physical or sexual abuse, and marital discord can be risk factors, as well. The list of potential pain risk factors goes on and on.

While some of these risk factors, such as smoking, obesity, and alcohol abuse, seem to be accepted in relation to heart disease, the acceptance by physicians and psychologists of these pain risk factors in cases of musculoskeletal pain is much less clear. Why is that?

PAIN AND BELIEF SYSTEMS

Like religions and political parties, the societies we live in have belief systems. What we believe affects how we look at the world and make decisions about things that happen within it. This discussion may be becoming too philosophical, but it boils down to two central questions that I would ask family doctors and medical specialists who are assessing patients experiencing painful conditions.

The first question is "Do you believe that pain can be caused or worsened by physical, environmental, social, and/or psychological factors?" The second question is "Do you believe that changes in patients' ergonomic, social, and/or psychological circumstances can help patients to improve and eventually even potentially completely recover from painful conditions?"

Most doctors' answer to the first question would be "Yes, I believe that pain can be caused or worsened by social and psychological factors." I don't think, however, that more than 50 percent of doctors actually believe in their hearts that trying to help their patients tackle their psychological and social problems can help patients overcome painful conditions. And this is the big issue. If M.D.s—and surely they are not alone—don't believe that psychological and social factors may matter in the resolution of their patients' back pain, migraine headaches, painful swallowing, or fibromyalgia symptoms, then they are not going to make major efforts to influence these issues in their practices. Their belief systems will not allow it.

MIND–BODY EDUCATION

But let's not just blame doctors. Medical school education is full of attempts to link health with social, economic, and environmental determinants. But that is not enough, or maybe it is already too late. Educating children about their health and how mind-body issues work is what is truly needed in society.

Many of my patients started to recognize the effects that their life circumstances could have on their pain only later on in life, when they were adults. Lloyd did not recognize that work- and stress-related issues could be influencing his neck pain until he had his first heart attack, and even then he wasn't so clear about the link. Helen realized the effects of stress only when deeply immersed in the pain of her fibromyalgia syndrome. Why does it take us so much time to recognize these relationships? It is because we aren't taught enough about the effects of feelings on health in grade school. But let's not complain. Let's try to explain.

Kids learn in school about sexuality, condoms, the pill, and how the body works. But do they learn that if they are worried and father is beating up mother, they may become stressed and experience a headache? Do they learn that if they are experiencing headaches or neck or back pain, it is worth talking about what is going on in their life, perhaps even before taking the over-the-counter pain medication? Maybe after Johnny discusses the bullying that he is experiencing, his body can relax, squeeze fewer neck muscles, and squirt less adrenaline into his system. Less acid may also be released into his stomach, and its lining may become less irritated.

We must teach children the warning signals of stress-related discomforts such as headaches, nausea, a sense of generally feeling unwell, neck or back tension, and tummy pain. They can then figure out for themselves what is going on or at least talk to their parents about their issues. They can learn how to be their own pain detectives. When I have discussed these concepts with teachers, they are usually very excited about them. But their implementation needs buy-in from school boards and school board parents, who themselves may need education about these pain-related topics.

MULTIPRONGED ATTACK

The previous chapters have outlined that there is not just one way to control or heal a painful condition. It takes a multipronged attack. As the pain explanation and treatment diagram used to help a number of patients in the stories indicates, a combined approach that looks at multiple physical, psychological, and social factors is usually required. It is indeed not easy to be a patient when so many individuals may be vying for their attention. Besides the doctor, there is a multitude of practitioners who regularly treat all kinds of musculoskeletal pain: physiotherapists, chiropractors, massage therapists, osteopaths, orthotists, pedorthists, acupuncturists, dieticians, naturopaths, occupational therapists, trainers, coaches, kinesiologists, social workers, and psychologists. The different types of medical doctors include anesthetists, physiatrists, rheumatologists, neurosurgeons, orthopedic surgeons, sports medicine physicians, and family physicians. I may have missed a few.

Any one of these individuals may be involved at one pain point or another. All may have tried to help the types of patients described in this book, via manual therapy, electrical stimulation, acupuncture, manipulation of various joints, medications, injections, and exercises. How did my patients choose which practitioner to go to? It is so hard to know who is the right person to see. I can't advocate one treatment as being vastly superior to another. I am, however, reminded of the expression that if you hand a carpenter a hammer, everything she looks at becomes a nail. That is, if one therapist performs a particular technique such as manipulation or injection, she may perform it exclusively, without suggesting other treatments.

Looking at the big picture—the history, the physical examination, and any laboratory or imaging tests deemed necessary—is still the only way to start. Finding out what the physical issues are, analyzing them, and assessing what other issues may be layered on top—that is really the only way to evaluate and treat a person's painful condition. Unfortunately, as the stories in this book show, there are no treatment shortcuts.

It takes time for key issues to rise to the top. And, even if important childhood, stress-related, or other psychological issues are discovered, medical investigations to rule out myriad possible diseases are always required. Only then can one safely pursue the multiple traditional and alternative treatments available today.

DISABILITY INSURANCE, LEGAL MATTERS

Some of the patients discussed, like Tyra and Mandy, were not working because of their pain or fatigue. They were receiving disability benefits from a long-term disability insurance plan that their employers had paid into for many years. Long-term disability insurance is a wonderful concept. If you are unable to work because of illness, the insurance company pays a large percentage of your salary so that you can still take care of your living expenses.

Insurance companies are great if you have a serious condition such as a stroke, spinal cord injury, or amputation, but they can be less client-friendly when it's a question of the types of musculoskeletal conditions described in *The Pain Detective* (e.g., back pain, fibromyalgia syndrome, chronic fatigue). This is another situation where belief systems "clash and burn." A colleague of mine has a leg disability that prevents him from running. As a doctor, he feels that no disability should prevent a person from working at a job. That is his belief system. Another colleague once told me, "Dr. F., I just don't believe that fibromyalgia syndrome can be disabling." That is her belief system. You can imagine how doctors' beliefs and attitudes affect, therefore, the delicate area of disability.

As part of their regular medical practice, doctors are asked daily by insurance companies whether or not a given patient qualifies for disability benefits—more specifically, whether or not the patient can work. I am sure that insurance companies would say that they want to be fair evaluators of their clients' conditions. And that is likely true. But insurance companies are also not in business to hand out money. Sometimes they will direct a client to a particular doctor whose "belief system" is that fibromyalgia syndrome is not disabling. An independent medical evaluation report will then read, "Ms. X can return to work. Her pain is disturbing her, but it is not disabling her." And the dilemmas and conflicts build. Another physician, who believes that more severe forms of fibromyalgia syndrome can be disabling, writes a second report at the request of a lawyer, indicating that Ms. X cannot return to work for the time being. And so it goes. Ultimately, the belief system battles affect primarily the patient, but the spillover to friends and family members is palpable, often in a sad, disheartening way.

The real tragedy is that, instead of evaluating the sources of the patient's disability, doctors spend too much energy helping patients "fight the system." There are obviously no quick solutions in situations like these, but getting to the root of the problem, not blaming the patient, and truly practicing mind-body medicine while simultaneously addressing physical, psychological, and social concerns can bring about positive results. Many of the stories told in this book reflect the success of this approach.

Pain Management, Outside the Box

It is time to think inside and outside the box when treating a patient with a persistent painful condition. When Bing Thom, an architect, saw the inaccessible waterfront of downtown Fort Worth, Texas, he asked himself, "What can be designed to bring the water to the people?" He proposed a brave new idea to create a bypass channel, and suddenly people could live on Forth Worth canals where they could not have lived before. Many other architects saw the same geographical setting and proposed designs that just maintained the status quo. The term "chronic pain," which I have used very little in this book but which is out there in society, is like the inaccessible waterfront of Fort Worth. If we do not address the sometimes complex psychological and social factors that may accompany pain, then potentially salvageable pain situations will go nowhere. If people can be helped to identify the physical and social issues that relate to their pain, then healing can occur and new treatment channels will be created. But, as in Texas, it takes community resources for this to happen. The services of physicians, physiotherapists, psychologists, and all the other musculoskeletal specialists previously noted, treating in a coordinated fashion, are required to allow such positive results to come to fruition.

Right now the average physician and patient do not have these types of practitioners at their easy disposal. Multidisciplinary pain centers that treat patients with painful conditions can be effective, but they are not prevalent, and they usually work with the most complex cases. All patients deserve a comprehensive treatment plan for their painful condition, but it is not common for them to receive one.

Conclusion

It is time to rein the horses in and head for home. There is no more time for doom and gloom. It is time to celebrate the hopeful stories told and the successes achieved. Maybe Rod Stewart did inspire me to choose "Every Ache Tells a Story" as part of the book's title; I will never really know. But I do know that the lessons learned from my patients' health journeys are powerful, thought provoking, and inspiring.

I have watched how deep emotional hurt, experienced by a patient as a child or as an adult, can influence how that patient's injured muscles and ligaments recover. I have read and written about scientists' observation that animal and human wounds recover more slowly when they occur in a stressed environment and that expressing deep emotions may reverse or improve this process. I have seen people come to grips with issues that they have been struggling with for years, with a subsequent positive effect on their pain condition.

Mind-body medicine is not some new-age concept practiced by a fringe element. It is a practice that we all know makes sense and fits with established principles of health, immunology, psychology, and physiology. It is just so hard to practice. So much of its success relies on experience and on having enough time to carry out the approaches outlined. It is hard to get it all right. And you end up falling down many times while trying to get it right. Not every patient described in this book does succeed at the end, because life does not work that way.

Every aspect of the pain explanation and treatment diagram cannot be addressed and attacked all at once. As I have stressed to my patients, "Let's string together a few sleep-filled instead of sleepless nights, a few days of increased exercise, a few hours of fewer cigarettes, chocolate bars, and beers, and we have a chance of slowly easing this pain problem. Let's identify those pain risk factors, the ones that squirt out buckets of adrenaline, and we can come up with a successful plan of attack."

FINAL WORDS

To the pain sufferer: Keep despair to a minimum. Analyze. Don't blame yourself. Recognize the hope in your situation; see the light at the end of the dark tunnel.

To the loved one of the pain sufferer: Support. Provide appropriate feedback. Try to understand.

To the reader who is just a "regular person": May these stories inspire you to learn more about yourself and the way your health interacts with your family, work, and community.

To the health care professional: Try to be part of a treatment team, however hard that is to achieve.

No pain, no gain? Untrue. If in pain, can you make gains? Yes. But your mind and body have to want to get better. And even then it is hard work. But rewarding.

Go. Good luck.

APPENDIX

Pain Explanation and Treatment Diagram

Hillel M. Finestone, MD
Physical Medicine and Rehabilitation

Name: _____

Date: _____

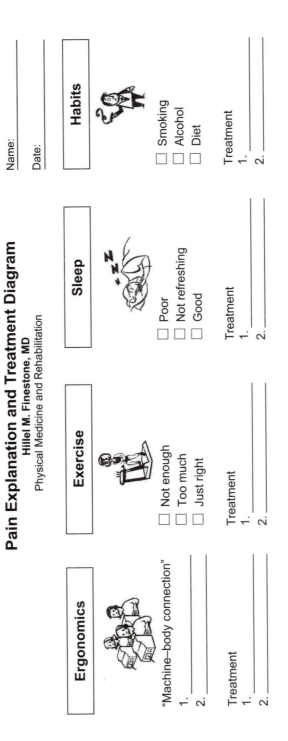

Ergonomics

"Machine—body connection"

1. _____
2. _____

Treatment
1. _____
2. _____

Exercise

☐ Not enough
☐ Too much
☐ Just right

Treatment
1. _____
2. _____

Sleep

☐ Poor
☐ Not refreshing
☐ Good

Treatment
1. _____
2. _____

Habits

☐ Smoking
☐ Alcohol
☐ Diet

Treatment
1. _____
2. _____

Other things that can affect, worsen or aggravate painful conditions – in anyone:

1. Life in general
2. Financial problems
3. Stress/anger/fear/nightmares
4. History of physical abuse
5. History of sexual abuse
6. Alcoholism (you or your family)
7. _____
8. _____

Treatment

1. _____
2. _____

Diagnosis

What I DO think your problems(s) is/are:

1. _____
2. _____
3. _____

What I DON'T think your problem(s) is/are:

☐ Bones ☐ Nerves ☐ Joints

How can stress affect, worsen, aggravate or cause pain? "Mind–body connection"

1. Adrenaline is squeezed into your bloodstream, your heart rate increases, your muscles tense up, and you sweat more. Your pain then increases and becomes more intense.
2. When you are injured, any stress that you feel can make the injury and the pain worse.
3. Relieving stress may relieve pain.

INDEX

About the Author

HILLEL M. FINESTONE, M.D. is a specialist in Physical Medicine and Rehabilitation (Physiatrist) at Bruyère Continuing Care, and Medical Director of the Stroke Rehabilitation Program at Élisabeth-Bruyère Hospital. He is also an Associate Professor on the faculty of medicine at the University of Ottawa. Dr. Finestone is a Fellow of the American Academy of Physical Medicine and Rehabilitation, a Fellow of the American Association of Neuromuscular and Electrodiagnostic Medicine, and a Fellow of the Royal College of Physicians and Surgeons of Canada. He has been interviewed by the BBC and Reuters News Service and featured in *USA Today,* the *New York Post,* and dozens of other newspapers and magazines in the United States, Canada, Europe, and the Middle East.

About the Series Editor

JULIE SILVER, M.D., is Assistant Professor, Harvard Medical School, Department of Physical Medicine and Rehabilitation, and is on the medical staff at Brigham and Women's, Massachusetts General, and Spaulding Rehabilitation Hospitals in Boston, Massachusetts. Dr. Silver has authored, edited, or co-edited more than a dozen books, including medical textbooks and consumer health guides. She is also the Chief Editor of Books at Harvard Health Publications. Dr. Silver has won many awards, including the American Medical Writers Association Solimene Award for Excellence in Medical Writing and the prestigious Lane Adams Quality of Life Award from the American Cancer Society. Silver is active teaching healthcare providers how to write and publish, and she is the founder and director of an annual seminar facilitated by the Harvard Medical School Department of Continuing Education, "Publishing Books, Memoirs, and Other Creative Nonfiction."